The

BIRTH PARTNER'S

Quick Reference Guide and Planner

Essential Labor and Childbirth
Information for Partners and Helpers

PENNY SIMKIN
with Katie Rohs

FAIR WINDS

PREFACE

This book is for those parents-to-be, loved ones, and doulas who will accompany a pregnant person through labor and birth. While the role is exciting, it can also be a bit scary if you don't know how to be helpful. We intend that this guide will give you the confidence and skills to be a positive part of the new parent's birth memory. Congratulations!

—Penny & Katie

Brimming with creative inspiration, how-to projects, and useful information to enrich your everyday life, Quarto Knows is a favorite destination for those pursuing their interests and passions. Visit our site and dig deeper with our books into your area of interest: Quarto Creates, Quarto Cooks, Quarto Homes, Quarto Lives, Quarto Drives, Quarto Explores, Quarto Gifts, or Quarto Kids.

© 2020 Quarto Publishing Group USA Inc.
Text © 2013, 2018, and 2020 Penny Simkin

First Published in 2019 by The Harvard Common Press, an imprint of The Quarto Group, 100 Cummings Center, Suite 265-D, Beverly, MA 01915, USA.
T (978) 282-9590 F (978) 283-2742 QuartoKnows.com

The Harvard Common Press titles are also available at discount for retail, wholesale, promotional, and bulk purchase. For details, contact the Special Sales Manager by email at specialsales@quarto.com or by mail at The Quarto Group, Attn: Special Sales Manager, 100 Cummings Center, Suite 265-D, Beverly, MA 01915, USA.

24 23 22 21 20   1 2 3 4 5

ISBN: 978-1-55832-977-5

Digital edition published in 2020

The content for this book appeared in the previously published *The Birth Partner, 7th Edition* (The Harvard Common Press 2018).

Library of Congress Cataloging-in-Publication Data available

Design: Sporto
Illustration: Gayle Isabelle Ford

Printed in China

CONTENTS

CHAPTER 1

The Last Weeks of Pregnancy 004

CHAPTER 2

Getting Into Labor 016

CHAPTER 3

Moving Through the Stages of Labor 028

CHAPTER 4

Comfort Measures for Labor 053

CHAPTER 5

Strategies for Challenging Variations in Normal Labor ... 086

CHAPTER 6

Tests, Technologies, Interventions, and Procedures 101

CHAPTER 7

Complications in Late Pregnancy, Labor, or Afterward 123

CHAPTER 8

Medications for Pain During Labor 138

CHAPTER 9

The First Days Postpartum 158

Labor and Birth Planners 180

Recommended Resources 190

Index 196

CHAPTER 1

The Last Weeks of Pregnancy

YOUR ROLE AS BIRTH PARTNER BEGINS before the pregnant person is in labor. During the last weeks of pregnancy, you can learn about labor, encourage the pregnant person to continue good health habits, help with last-minute preparations for the baby and for labor itself, and figure out the role you will play as birth partner. You can prepare for your role through self-examination, discussions with the pregnant person, gathering information, and practicing comfort measures.

This is also the time for you both to make many important decisions about the birth and to discuss them with the caregiver. If you attend childbirth classes and go to prenatal checkups, you will not only become informed, but also meet the doctors or midwives and become more comfortable in your role. You can also get advice and reassurance about anything causing anxiety or uncertainty for either of you.

Early in pregnancy, it seems that nine months are forever and there is plenty of time to do everything that has to be done. It is all too easy, especially for busy people, to postpone "getting into" the pregnancy. Now, suddenly, the baby is almost due. Time has flown by. As the pregnant person's birth partner, you realize you are being counted on to help them through childbirth. Do you feel ready? Can you help? What do you know about labor? Do you know what to do when? What should you do now to get ready for the baby? The last months of pregnancy are a perfect time to learn these things, but you had better start right away—a month or two before the due date is truly the "last minute," especially as many babies arrive early.

GETTING READY FOR LABOR

If you haven't already done the things described in the following pages, try to do so a few weeks before the due date or at least before labor starts.

Visit the Pregnant Person's Caregiver (Doctor or Midwife)

If you have not yet met the caregiver, this visit may be more important than you think—for both you and the caregiver. Even a brief meeting helps establish for the caregiver that you are an important person in the pregnant person's life. Although a substitute caregiver (another partner in the group practice) may actually attend the birth, this meeting still provides you the opportunity to ask questions, get a feel for what doctors and midwives do, and play a more active role.

Preregister at the Hospital

If you're having a hospital birth, you should preregister, which involves obtaining, reading, and signing pre-admission forms and a medical consent form. By registering in advance, you save time and avoid confusion when you arrive with the pregnant person in labor.

Consider Having a Doula Help You Both During Labor

Why consider a doula? Childbirth is intense, demanding, unpredictable, and painful, and it can last for a few hours to 24, 36, or even more. Even if you are well prepared, you and the pregnant person may find it difficult to apply your classroom learning in the real situation. If you are not well prepared, all the challenges of labor are baffling and anxiety producing.

Of course, you will have a nurse and a doctor or midwife who are likely to be kind and caring, but they will probably be very busy with the clinical aspects of the birth, which are their highest priority. Hospital nurses and midwives rarely remain in the room throughout labor, as they must take breaks, perform duties outside the room and are often taking care of more than one laboring patient at a time. They work in shifts, so over the course of labor, several different professionals are likely to be involved in each laboring person's care. Doctors rely on the nurses to manage the labor, with phone reports as necessary, and they may briefly visit from time to time and will come if problems arise during labor. And, of course, they are there for the birth.

One of the most positive developments in maternity care is the addition of the birth doula, who guides and supports women and their partners continuously through labor and birth. The doula usually meets with you in advance, is on call for you, arrives at your home or the hospital when you need her, and remains with you continuously, with few breaks, until after the baby is born. The doula is trained and experienced in providing emotional support, physical comfort, and nonclinical advice. They draw on their knowledge and experience as they reassure, encourage, comfort, and empathize with the laboring person. The doula also works with the partner, guiding and assisting you on how to help, suggesting when to use particular positions, the bath or shower, and specific comfort measures.

A doula cannot and does not take over your role as the birth partner because you know the birthing person better and love them and the baby as no one else does. But there are many times when the person giving birth needs more than one helper in labor, and the partner needs reassurance, advice, and help, too.

Besides helping the laboring person, a doula can help you in these ways:

- Guide you in applying the information you learned in childbirth class to the more stressful and unpredictable labor situation.
- Relieve you so you can get a meal, a nap, or just a break during a long or all-night labor.
- Bring beverages, hot packs, or ice for the laboring person so you do not have to leave to do so.

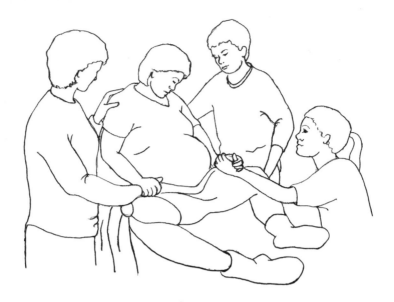

- Reassure you if you are worried about the laboring person's well-being. The doula's experience provides perspective, which can keep you from misinterpreting normal reactions to labor as signs that something is wrong or that the laboring person is not coping well.
- Help you understand what the laboring person might be feeling and interpret the signs of labor progress to you.
- Provide support and help you participate more confidently, if you do not feel comfortable as the laboring person's only constant source of support, by making sure the laboring person's needs are met.
- By getting to know the two of you before the birth, the doula can discover your priorities, fears, and concerns and help develop strategies to deal with them.
- Photograph or videotape the two of you during labor and birth or all three (or more!) of you afterward. Check hospital policies on this.

Doulas do not make decisions for you or project personal preferences on you, but rather help you get the information you need to make good decisions. A doula's goal is to help the laboring person have a satisfying birth as they define it.

One partner described the doula this way: "She was like my big sister—ready, willing, and able to help me do the best job I could. She showed me how to rub Mary's back, reminded us to try the lunge (see page 69), and got me a bagel when I was really hungry. She kept encouraging us. She seemed so confident. A lot of the time, both she and I were helping Mary. I was holding her during the contractions, and our doula was pressing on Mary's back and helping her breathe in rhythm. Our doula even gave me a shoulder rub in the middle of the night. She never left except to go to the bathroom. Without her, the birth wouldn't have been as great for both Mary and me. The doula helped me do a better job."

Numerous scientific trials have compared birth outcomes of women who had doulas and those who did not. In very "high-tech" hospitals with high cesarean and induction rates, women attended by doulas had fewer forceps and vacuum-extractor deliveries and fewer cesareans. They did not need to use as much pain medication. Also, women attended by a doula were more likely to report birth experiences that were satisfying versus those who did not have a doula. Although a doula cannot guarantee a normal or an easy labor, statistics show that having a doula results in less need for major labor interventions. Chapter 3 describes what doulas do to help during each phase of labor.

There are many organizations that train and certify birth doulas, with different methods of training and requirements for certification. When choosing your doula, it's important to consider the doula's training. DoulaMatch.net has a comprehensive guide to evaluating doula-certifying organizations, which can help guide your selection.

We agree with DoulaMatch.net's suggestions for choosing a doula trained by a high-quality training organization. They are reprinted here with permission of Doula-Match (see Recommended Resources, page 190) for more information:

- A comprehensive doula-training program, which includes requirements for in-person classroom work, self-study, and practicum work with minimum hours for each requirement clearly stated.
- Clearly defined requirements for a doula's education.
- Demonstrated doula work experience.
- Good evaluations from clients and health care providers.
- Periodic recertification.
- Documented continuing education.
- A publicly available code of ethics outlining the doula's ethical responsibilities to clients.
- A publicly available standards of practice defining the doula's scope and limits of practice.
- A grievance procedure allowing consumers, colleagues, or care providers to lodge an objection against the organization's doula if they violate the organization's standards of practice or code of ethics. The goal of the grievance procedure is to uncover the facts of the objection and seek resolution for the injured parties or consequences for the doula, including revoking certification.

Costs of doula services vary greatly: In the United States, costs range from a few hundred dollars to as much as $2,500 or more in some large cities depending on the doula's experience. Some hospitals have volunteer or paid doulas available during labor, and some community agencies and charitable organizations employ doulas to care for clients for whom doula costs may be challenging. Some trained doulas offer low-cost services while gaining experience to apply for certification. Others offer free service to people in their own ethnic or religious communities. Some health insurers cover doula fees, and some clients can use health savings accounts to cover doula fees.

Choose and Meet with Your Doula

If you decide to have a doula, it is a good idea to start looking for one a few months before the baby is due; doulas are often fully booked for weeks or months in advance. Get referrals from your care provider, childbirth educator, or friends who have used a doula. You can also contact DONA International (DONA.org) and search their database of certified doulas or try DoulaMatch.net. Most doulas now have personal websites; take time to read their information and select three to four doulas to contact and interview. If the information isn't available on a website, ask whether the doula is available around your due date and what the fee is. If the fee is outside your budget, you can ask for a payment plan or sliding scale fee or ask for a referral to another doula. To ensure a good match, interview the doula in person.

There is usually no charge for the first get-acquainted interview with a doula, which usually lasts an hour or so. This interview is an opportunity for you to get to know the doula and for the doula to get to know you. It is important to choose a doula whose philosophy and approach are congruent with your desires for birth or who can unconditionally support your wishes for the birth. There are many lists online for questions to ask a doula, and we especially like those on the DONA.org website and on DoulaMatch.net. Some topics you might discuss:

- The doula's calendar around the pregnant person's due date (other clients due about the same time, plans to be out of town, unbreakable obligations)
- Backup arrangements (every doula should have reliable backup in case two clients are in labor at the same time, illness, or other unforeseen emergencies)
- The doula's training and certification and the reasons for choosing the training/certification organization
- The support included in the doula's package:
    - Number of prenatal visits
    - Type of postpartum support provided
    - Point at which the doula joins the client in labor
    - Time limits for in-person support, including what happens in the case of a long labor
- Type of phone, email, or text support the doula provides
- Payment arrangements and possibility of health insurance or health savings account reimbursement

Some doulas offer other services, such as private childbirth preparation, massage, birth-related counseling, placental encapsulation, breast-feeding help, or postpartum doula care. There usually are additional charges for these services.

Be Reachable by Phone—Always

You can never know when labor will start and you'll be needed. Both of you should carry a cell phone, charged and turned on, whenever you are not together. If your job takes you far away or out of cell phone range, check in with the pregnant person often and have someone else available when you are not. Make sure that person can be reached at all times, too, and will come to the laborer's aid, night or day, on very short notice.

Gather Necessary Supplies

Use the packing and supplies section of the Labor and Birth Planners, page 180, to track the supplies you will want to take to the hospital or birth center.

Encourage Regular Exercise

Regular exercise, such as walking, prenatal yoga, water aerobics, or swimming, helps maintain or improve a pregnant person's general fitness. Prenatal yoga is especially helpful in enabling relaxation during pain and developing one's inner resources for remaining calm during labor. Encourage the pregnant person to join a class. In addition, you or a friend might take walks or swim with them.

A few special exercises can be particularly helpful during late pregnancy and labor: squatting, pelvic rock on hands and knees (called cat-cow in yoga), and the pelvic floor contraction (Kegel) exercise. The information on the pelvic floor exercises includes instructions on whether and how to do this exercise.

SQUATTING

This may be very useful in helping the baby move down during the birthing stage. Ten squats per day, with heels on the floor and support (from you or using two doorknobs) lasting for up to 1 minute each, should increase the pregnant person's comfort and stamina with the position.

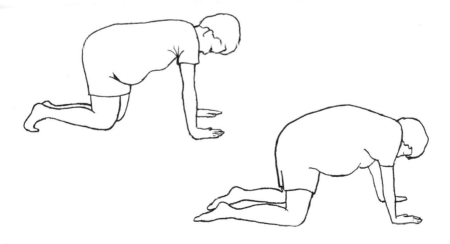

> **CAUTION:** If the pregnant person has joint problems in the ankles, knees, or hips or develops pain in these joints or in the pubic joint (in the middle below the abdomen), do not practice squatting.

A birth stool may give some of the same advantages as squatting, without stressing the joints in the legs. Consult the illustrations (page 74) to see how a partner supports a person while squatting.

PELVIC ROCK ON HANDS AND KNEES (CAT-COW)

During pregnancy, this exercise helps strengthen abdominal muscles, relieve low back pain, and improve circulation in the lower half of the body. During labor, the pelvic rock also helps relieve back pain and position the baby in the favorable OA (occiput anterior) position.

On hands and knees, the pregnant person should tuck the pelvis under while arching the back, for a slow count of five, and then return to normal briefly. While arching, one should feel the abdominal muscles working very hard but should do not hold one's breath. Repeat for a total of ten times per day (see illustrations, page 76).

PELVIC FLOOR CONTRACTIONS (KEGELS)

Many people (regardless of gender) can benefit from pelvic floor contraction exercises. These strengthen the muscles that support the pelvic organs, improve urinary and bowel control, and help prevent hemorrhoids as well as increase sexual pleasure. During pregnancy, having a good resting tension in the pelvic floor muscles protects against incontinence (involuntary loss of urine or stool) and pelvic organ prolapse. In childbirth, these toned muscles help the baby rotate and descend (see page 26). The laboring person's ability to relax these muscles in childbirth, especially in the second stage as they push the baby down the birth canal, greatly assists the birth. Having established healthy function and control of the pelvic floor muscles before childbirth can help restore function more quickly postpartum.

However, some people should not do pelvic floor strengthening exercises—those who already have very strong or tense pelvic floors. Endurance athletes or people who have had painful or traumatic experiences involving the pelvic floor probably should not do the strengthening exercises. If the pregnant person has tightness or pain in the pelvic floor, they would be wise to see a physical therapist who is a specialist on the pelvic floor. See Recommended Resources for a link to "Pelvic Floor Self-Assessment."

Because pelvic floor contraction exercises are important for everyone's lifelong general health, we describe the exercise in detail here.

Everyone (regardless of gender or age) performs the exercise in the same way. Contract by squeezing and lifting the pelvic floor muscles upward. Squeeze as you would if trying to keep from urinating or passing gas. Do five to ten quick contractions in a row. Now, hold a contraction for up to 10 seconds. You may find it difficult, at first, to do these longer holds, but your stamina will improve with practice. If the contraction seems to fade when you have not consciously let go, reengage your muscles to tighten again. After

10 seconds, let go and rest. Try another 10-second hold, but this time try not to contract the muscles in your legs, buttocks, or abdomen. Try also to do them without holding your breath.

Do ten 10-second pelvic floor contractions a day. You and the pregnant person can remind each other to do them while riding in the car or bus, waiting in line, or talking on the telephone. Or, do one or two while washing your hands after using the toilet.

Prepare and Review the Birth Plan

The birth plan is a written document that tells the caregiver and nurses which options are important to the birthing person, what their priorities are, any specific concerns, and how they want to be cared for during labor, birth, and the first few hours after the baby is born. The plan should reflect an awareness that medical needs could require a shift from the written choices, and it should include a Plan B—including preferences in case labor stalls or there are problems with the laboring person or the baby. Although most useful for birth in a hospital, where the nurses (and often the caregivers) do not know the pregnant person, a birth plan can help every couple, even those planning a home or birth-center birth, to think through their choices and priorities. And, because some planned out-of-hospital births require transfer to the hospital, a transfer plan is also a very good idea.

The birth plan is most useful when short and concise—one page is best; no more than two. We suggest using bulleted sentences or brief paragraphs, with any details that seem appropriate, for each of the relevant items that follow. Find out your hospital's and caregiver's usual practices before preparing your birth plan. If you both are comfortable with those practices, you don't have to list them. Only list preferences that differ from the usual care.

INTRODUCTION TO THE BIRTH PLAN

Your plan might begin with the following information:

- **Personal information (two or three sentences).** What does the pregnant person want the staff to know about them? For example, describe strongly held beliefs or preferences, relevant previous experiences with health care, trauma, fears, concerns, or other information that can help staff know them and treat them as an individual.
- **Message to staff.** Do the two of you want to express appreciation for any support, expertise, and assistance staff can provide to help you have a safe and satisfying birth experience? If you both want to be involved in decision-making regarding your care, say so here (see pages 101 and 102). Let the staff know you understand that labor sometimes requires flexibility and a change from your desired options by using phrases like, "as long as labor proceeds normally" or "unless medically indicated."
- **Making medical care decisions.** How do you like to make decisions as they relate to medical care? Assuming the situation does not require urgent action, do you and the laboring person want private time to discuss the situation and come to a decision? Do you prefer that the care provider offer recommendations you can accept or reject?
- **Support team.** Names of those on the support team who will attend the birth.

LABOR OPTIONS

The pregnant person can consider the following options for labor. To keep the plan brief, try to condense their wishes to general statements.

- Options include a preference to rely mainly on self-help and nondrug approaches to pain (see pages 54–64) or on pain medications or epidural block (see "Pain Medications Preference Scale," pages 145–146).
- Include general preference regarding use of procedures and interventions. Is the pregnant person okay with usual routines or using them only when medically necessary (see Chaper 6)?

BIRTH OPTIONS

The pregnant person can consider the following options for birth:

- Positions. Freedom to move and use a variety of positions or to lie on their back or in one position for long periods (see pages 169–176).
- Pushing techniques. Spontaneous, nondirected bearing down or prolonged breath holding and straining with directed pushing (see page 164).
- Perineal care. Warm compresses on the perineum and other measures to help relax and push effectively; preferences regarding episiotomy or avoiding episiotomy (see page 118). If the pregnant person has been doing perineal massage to improve the chances of an intact perineum, say so.

AFTER-BIRTH OPTIONS

The birthing person can consider the following options in postpartum care:

- Immediate care of the baby. Contact with the baby: immediate skin- to-skin contact with the birthing parent or removed to a warmer for initial procedures and wrapping; immediate or delayed umbilical cord clamping and cutting, for a few minutes or until it stops pulsating (see pages 161-162); routine suctioning or omitting suctioning baby's nose and mouth if baby is vigorous; immediate or delayed newborn routines (eye care, vitamin K, newborn exam, weighing, and so forth) until parents have boning time with the baby (see pages 51–52).
- Cord blood (public donation or private storage). You may choose to have placental blood extracted immediately after birth for future use in treating a variety of serious diseases. The cord blood may be donated to a blood bank for public access. Alternatively, it may be stored privately with a for-profit company at considerable cost to the family, where it is reserved for that family's use only. If you choose private storage, say so in your birth plan. To learn more about this option, see chapter 10, and Recommended Resources (page 190).
- Your presence. Whether you stay in the hospital with the postpartum parent and baby or return to visit each day.
- Feeding. Breastfeeding or formula-feeding.
- Circumcision. Yes or no if the baby is born with a penis (see page 167).

THE UNEXPECTED, OR PLAN B

The two of you should think through the possibility of extra challenges or complications, such as a long, exhausting labor or problems for the laboring person or baby. For safety or well-being, interventions may become necessary, and some of the preferences you list for a normal labor and birth may no longer be appropriate. Consider the following:

- Difficult labor or complications. Parents can leave all care decisions to the staff or they continue to participate in decision-making after receiving explanations of the situations and discussion of possible nonmedical and medical options, including waiting.

- Cesarean birth. Options to think about if a cesarean becomes necessary: degree of information the laboring person wants before and during surgery; presence of you, the doula or both; preferences about pain medications (any sedation that causes sleepiness, along with the epidural or spinal, during the surgery); contact with the baby after birth (skin to skin as soon as possible or wrapped in a blanket in the operating room or in recovery). If the baby needs to go to the intensive care nursery, do you go with the baby or stay with the birthing person? (A doula or other loved one can stay with the birthing person while you go to the nursery.) Does the birthing parent prefer to have sleep or sedative medications afterward for trembling and/or nausea or to wait to see if it is needed in order to remain awake and hold and nurse the baby (see chapter 9)?

- Premature or sick infant. Possible options: Involvement by both in the baby's care and feeding versus minimal contact; involvement in decision-making and explanations of the baby's problems, the procedures to be done, and possible options versus leaving care decisions entirely up to staff. If the baby cannot breast-feed, the birthing person tube-feeds or bottle-feeds the baby with expressed colostrum or (later) milk versus giving the baby formula. Once discharged, parents to receive resources for follow-up of the baby and support for parents.

- Stillbirth or death of the baby. Such a tragedy, as rare as it is, leaves the parents so stunned with grief it is almost impossible to make important decisions. Discuss this possibility together and think about how you and the pregnant person want the situation handled. You may want the opportunity to hold or dress your baby and say goodbye in private; save mementos such as the baby's clothing or blanket, some hand or footprints, or a lock of hair. Weeks or months after the death of a baby, the things that were done (or not done) at the time will be very important.

The 36-week prenatal appointment is a good time to give the birth plan to the doctor or midwife. It can then be placed in the pregnant person's hospital chart, where other staff will have access to it. Use the birth plan as a guide but be willing to accept changes if medically necessary.

PREPARING FOR LIFE WITH THE BABY

Following is a reminder list of some things to do before the baby is born. It is easier to do these things before the birth rather than afterward, when time and energy are limited.

Take a Baby Care and Safety Class

You'll want to learn about a newborn's temperament, capabilities, and needs; how they communicate needs; how to soothe newborn babies; diapering and bathing; guidelines for safe sleeping; how to tell whether a baby is sick; making your home safe for your baby; infant cardiopulmonary resuscitation (CPR); and more. Most hospitals and parent-support organizations offer such classes or can help you find them. If you can't take a class, get a good book on baby care (see Recommended Resources, page 190).

Gather Essential Supplies for the Baby

Is everything ready for the baby? Are the necessary supplies on hand? Use the packing and supplies section of the Labor and Birth Planners, page 180, to track your acquisition of the most necessary supplies.

Choose a Caregiver or Clinic for the Baby

The baby will need a medical caregiver (pediatrician, family doctor, naturopathic doctor, nurse practitioner, or health clinic) to provide well-baby care (routine checkups, immunizations) and to treat illnesses if they occur. Check the baby's health insurance plan for a list of preferred providers and get recommendations from friends, your childbirth educator, or the pregnant person's caregiver. Many parents make the baby's first doctor's appointment based on these recommendations or from information on the doctors' websites. However, some children's doctors provide opportunities for parents to meet them before making a selection, which allows you both to discover their views on topics important to you and determine whether you feel comfortable with them. The following are important considerations when choosing a caregiver. Check the list to narrow your choices for an interview:

- **Location of the office.** How far away is it? There is a real advantage to its being close to home. Traveling a long distance with a sick child can be nerve-wracking.
- **Practical considerations.** Is the caregiver covered by your health insurance? What are the caregiver's educational and professional qualifications? What are the fees? Who covers the practice when the caregiver is not available? At which hospital(s), if any, does the caregiver have privileges?
- **Questions to ask during the get-acquainted appointment.** If you have an opportunity to meet the doctor in advance, you might ask one or two questions about topics that are important to you, such as breastfeeding, infant sleep, immunizations, or starting solid foods.

- **Personal attributes.** Does this caregiver seem kind, competent, and caring? Is this someone whom both of you could trust with your baby's health care? Most importantly, is the caregiver's approach consistent with your values and beliefs regarding health and medical care?

Investigate Parent-Infant Classes or Peer-Support Groups

Classes and drop-in or online support groups for new parents are widely available. Consult your childbirth educator, doula, or caregiver for possibilities. Also, hospitals near you may offer new-parent groups. These classes and support groups provide information about child development, emotional needs of parents and infants, and discuss common problems. Parents learn exercises, songs, massage techniques, techniques for soothing crying babies, and games to play with their newborns. If it's convenient and appealing to you, attend the classes together. You may enjoy the opportunity to form new friendships and share your questions, concerns, and triumphs.

CHAPTER 2

Getting Into Labor

THE CLIMAX OF PREGNANCY—the birth of a baby—is an everyday miracle for the family, but just part of a day's work for the doctor, midwife, or nurse. For you, the birthing person, and those who love and support them, it is a deep and permanent memory. Your role as birth partner is to do as much as possible to *help make this birth experience a good memory for the person giving birth.* This birth is an event that will never be forgotten—including the good and the bad. The kind of care a person receives and the quality of support during labor make the difference in whether the birth experience is remembered with satisfaction and fulfillment or disappointment and sadness. This is where you come in. Being a birth partner—helping someone through labor and birth—is clearly a challenge, but it is a challenge that people like you meet all the time.

To be a good birth partner, you need:

- A bond of love or friendship with, and feelings of commitment and responsibility toward, the birthing person.
- Familiarity with the birthing person's personal preferences and quirks, the little things that are soothing and relaxing, and the things that may be irritating or worrying.
- A commitment to help continuously throughout labor, either by yourself or with the help of a doula or other supportive person.
- Knowledge of what to expect—the physical process of labor, the procedures and interventions commonly used during labor, and when these procedures and interventions are necessary and when they are optional.
- An understanding of the emotional side of labor—the emotional needs of laboring people and the changing emotions usually experienced as labor progresses.
- Practical knowledge of how to help in various specific situations—what to do when. A trained doula can help with this and the two preceding points.
- Flexibility to adapt to the laboring person's changing needs during labor—leading by following. How you help, and how much you help, are determined by the laboring person's needs and responses at the time.

The next few chapters cover the normal birth process and explain what happens, how the birthing person is likely to respond, what the caregiver does, and how you can help. These chapters also discuss situations that are particularly difficult for the laboring person and, therefore, particularly challenging for the birth partner, too. Read these chapters in advance and use them as an on-the-spot guide during labor.

Everyone wonders how to tell whether a pregnant person is in labor. Even those with experience cannot usually identify exactly when labor starts. Often the labor "sneaks" up with unclear, on-again-off-again signs—like an orchestra tuning up before a performance. Over the course of many hours or days, the signs intensify, and you both come to realize that something is different—this is *it*! Step by step, the birthing person becomes mentally and physically more ready for the coordinated effort that eventually results in the birth of the baby. It is normal to experience a period of uncertainty and questioning while awaiting clear signs that labor has truly started.

As long as the two of you eventually put the pieces together, it usually doesn't matter if the labor is vague at the beginning. There is almost always plenty of time, once labor clearly starts, to get to the hospital or birth center or settle in for a home birth. Occasionally, however, a pregnant person is caught by surprise and goes into labor earlier or more suddenly than anticipated. Because of this possibility, you will want to be able to tell the difference between the tuning up, or prelabor, and the real thing, progressing labor.

This chapter helps you recognize when labor truly starts. It explains how labor begins physically and emotionally and describes the role you should play as birth partner.

THE DIFFERENCE BETWEEN PRELABOR AND LABOR

Labor is the process by which someone gives birth to a baby and a placenta. It usually follows hours or days of prelabor contractions, which are shorter, less frequent, and less intense than labor contractions. In prelabor, the cervix begins to soften and thin and is preparing to open once labor is established. The labor process involves the following:

1. Contractions of the uterus, the largest and strongest muscle in the pregnant body. These build in intensity and frequency over time.
2. Softening (ripening), thinning (effacement), and opening (dilation) of the cervix.
3. Breaking of the bag of waters (the membranes or amniotic sac) surrounding the baby and the release of water (amniotic fluid), either as a leak or a gush.
4. Rotation and molding of the baby's head and tucking of the chin, to fit into the pelvis.
5. Descent of the baby out of the uterus and through the birth canal (pelvis and vagina) to the outside.
6. Birth of the placenta.
7. The first hours when parents and baby ideally stay together with the baby, skin to skin with a parent, feeding, and getting to know each other.

Normally, labor does not begin until both the pregnant parent and baby are ready—between 38 and 42 weeks of pregnancy. The last weeks prepare the pregnant person physically and psychologically to give birth and breastfeed and nurture a baby. During this time, the baby acquires the "final touches" preparing for the stress of labor and adaptation to life outside the uterus. It is the baby who usually initiates the labor, by producing and secreting the hormones that begin the chain of events leading to the steps just listed.

In 2017, about one in ten U.S. babies was born prematurely, before being really ready. Premature birth may be due to conditions in the pregnant person—infection, high stress, poverty, heavy smoking, poor nutrition, drug use, or unknown reasons that override the mechanisms normally initiated by the baby. Multiple pregnancies (twins, triplets, and more) and some fetal abnormalities are other causes.

Very few babies are born after 42 weeks (post-term). The belief among most leaders is that there are few benefits to waiting. This has led to widespread polices of induction.

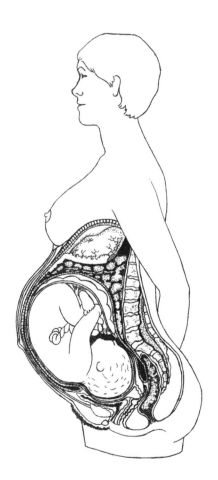

HOW LONG WILL LABOR LAST?

It is impossible to predict how long any particular labor will last. A perfectly normal labor can take between 2 and 24 hours following hours or days of prelabor. Many factors influence the length of labor:

- Whether this is a first or later baby
- The condition of the cervix (soft and thin or firm and thick) when labor contractions begin
- The size of the baby, particularly the head, in relation to the size of the pregnant person's pelvis
- The presentation and position of the baby's head within the pregnant person's body
- The strength and frequency of the contractions
- The pregnant person's emotional state—if lonely, frightened, or angry, labor may be slower than when the person is confident, content, and calm
- *Presentation* refers to the part of the baby—top of the head (the vertex), brow, face, buttocks, feet, shoulders—that is lowest in the uterus. The vertex almost always *presents* first; problems may occur in delivery if any other part of the baby presents first. *Position* refers to the placement of the presenting part within the pregnant person's pelvis. The most common positions are:
- **OA (occiput anterior):** The back of the baby's head (the occiput) points toward the pregnant person's front (anterior).
- **OT (occiput transverse):** The back of the baby's head points toward the pregnant person's side (transverse).
- **OP (occiput posterior):** The back of the baby's head points toward the pregnant person's back (posterior).

Although babies can and usually do change position during labor and during the pushing (second) stage, at birth, the OA position is much more common than OT or OP. When the baby is in the OP position in labor, with the back of their head toward the pregnant person's back, labor is sometimes prolonged, and the laboring person may experience intense backache. There are many other reasons for back pain in labor, however (see page 96). Do not assume the baby is OP just because the laboring person has back pain.

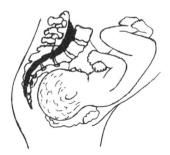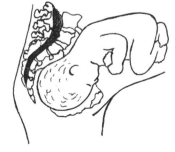

A baby in OA (occiput anterior) position (left) and OP (occiput posterior) position (right)

SIGNS OF LABOR

How will you know labor has started? A few clues can usually help you recognize labor long before the birth is imminent. It is equally important, though, to be able to tell when the pregnant person is not in labor. There is nothing more frustrating or disappointing for someone than thinking labor has begun and discovering, after a trip to the caregiver or hospital, that the cervix is not opening (or dilating), which is the most important sign of labor (which results in going home to wait). The best way to avoid this is to know the signs of labor (see table, pages 21 and 22) and how to interpret them. Some signs are clearer than others. They are categorized as Possible Signs, Prelabor Signs, and Positive Signs.

- **Possible Signs (tuning up):** Without other signs, these signs are not clear enough to get excited about. They can fool and confuse a pregnant person because they feel different from what they were feeling earlier. However, unlike the Positive Signs, they do not indicate that the cervix is dilating and that labor has started. Rather, Possible Signs indicate the body is getting ready for labor. These signs may continue, on and off, for days or even weeks, before the cervix begins to dilate. We do not recommend that you or the pregnant person go away on a trip when these signs are present because, at any time, they might turn the corner into labor. If the pregnant person has had a rapid labor with a previous birth, they should be particularly alert to the Possible Signs, as these might be all the signs that occur before suddenly going into another rapid labor.
- **Prelabor Signs:** These are more important than Possible Signs, but real labor could still be hours, or even days, away.
- **Positive Signs:** These are the most certain signs that labor has truly started—that is, the cervix is dilating.

If you know the significance of these signs, chances are very good you will correctly interpret what is happening. Sometimes, though, couples need a caregiver's help to figure out whether the pregnant person is really in labor. You should certainly call your caregiver if there are any Prelabor or Positive signs before 37 weeks, as they could indicate the onset of premature labor.

SIGNS AND SYMPTOMS	COMMENTS
• **Possible Signs (late pregnancy changes)** • Vague nagging backache causing restlessness— a need to keep changing positions • Several soft bowel movements—sometimes accompanied by flu-like "sick" feelings • Cramps, similar to menstrual cramps, that come and go; the discomfort may extend to the thighs • Unusual burst of energy resulting in great activity (cleaning, organizing)— termed the "nesting urge" • **Prelabor Signs** • Nonprogressing contractions—that is, contractions that continue without changing; they do not become longer, stronger, and closer together over time. They sometimes last for hours and subside before restarting. These are prelabor, or Braxton Hicks, contractions (see "'False' Labor, or Prelabor," page 23, and "Timing Contractions," page 26). • Water leaks, resulting in a trickle (not a gush) of fluid from the vagina (see "If the Bag of Waters Breaks Before Labor Begins," page 22.) • Blood-tinged mucus discharge ("show" or mucus plug) may be released from the vagina before labor; more likely to occur once there are other Positive Signs (see following); laboring person continues passing this discharge off and on throughout labor • **Positive Signs** • Progressing contractions—that is, contractions that become longer, stronger, and closer together over time. These usually continue until it is time to push. Some laboring people having second or subsequent babies, however, have periods of progressing contractions that come and go over a few days before they settle into a continuous pattern (see page 26 for instructions on timing contractions).	• Different from the fatigue-related backache common during pregnancy • When this sign accompanies others, it is probably associated with an increase in hormone-like substances in the bloodstream (prostaglandins). These substances soften and thin the cervix and stimulate bowel activity. By itself, this symptom may be due to digestive upset. • May be associated with prostaglandin action and early contractions • May go away and return several times over weeks or progress steadily to Positive Signs • Accomplishes softening and thinning of the cervix, preparing the cervix to begin dilating • Should not be perceived as unproductive • Usually not painful, but may be tiring or discouraging if they continue for many hours • Leaking fluid occurs before labor in about 2 of every 10 labors. • A signal: call and report to caregiver • Associated with thinning of the cervix • May occur days before other signs or not until after progressing contractions have begun • A discharge, often mistaken for show, may also appear within a day after a pelvic exam or sexual intercourse and is not a sign of labor. Show is pink or red; the discharge after a pelvic exam or sex tends to be brownish. • The cervix is very likely to be opening if they have 12 to 15 contractions in a row that are consistently 1 minute long, occur 3 or fewer minutes apart, and feel painful or "very strong." • It is an even clearer sign if these contractions are combined with a "show" (blood-tinged discharge). • The laboring person cannot be distracted from these contractions. • Contractions may be felt in the abdomen, back, or both. • Often associated with rapid labor • The bag of waters usually breaks in late labor. Rupture of the membranes with a gush occurs before other signs of labor in only 1 or 2 out of 10 labors.

CAUTION: If the pregnant person is less than 37 weeks' pregnant and experiences four or more noticeable contractions in 1 hour for more than 2 hours, combined with any of the other Possible, Prelabor, or Positive signs of labor, they should consult their caregiver. This might be premature labor, which can sometimes be stopped if caught early. The caregiver may ask them to go in to be checked or to first drink some fluids and lie down to see if the contractions stop. If the contractions don't stop, they'll be asked to go the caregiver's office or the hospital to determine whether it is preterm labor. Catching this early often means stopping it. If the pregnant person is beyond 37 weeks and the pregnancy is normal, wait for the Positive Signs before calling the caregiver.

IF THE BAG OF WATERS BREAKS BEFORE LABOR BEGINS

If the pregnant person's membranes rupture—if water leaks or gushes from the vagina—before labor begins, make the following observations to report to the caregiver:

1. *The amount* of fluid: Is it a trickle, a leak, or a gush? A "leak" is a squirt that occurs when a pregnant person changes position; about 2 in 10 labors begin this way. A "gush" is an uncontrollable heavy flow that may start with a popping feeling. About 1 or 2 in 10 labors begins this way.
2. **The *color* of the fluid:** Normally, the fluid is clear. If it is brownish or greenish, the baby may have had a bowel movement (passed meconium), which happens when a baby is stressed in the uterus. Such stress is caused by a temporary lack of oxygen. While usually not serious, the caregiver may want to check the baby's well-being.
3. **The *odor* of the fluid:** Normally, the fluid is practically odorless. If it has a foul smell, there may be an infection within the uterus, which could spread to the baby.

This information helps the caregiver plan what to do next—whether to stay home, with precautions, or go to the hospital or caregiver's office so some of the fluid can be collected and tested to determine whether it is amniotic fluid or something else (liquid mucus or urine). To collect fluid from the vagina, the caregiver uses a sterile speculum and a sterile swab. This test is important if the status of the membranes is not clear.

One concern with ruptured membranes is whether the pregnant person is a carrier of Group B streptococcus, a type of bacteria present in vaginal secretions of about one-third of people. If so, the caregiver may want to start treatment with antibiotics and, if labor does not begin spontaneously, induce labor in a matter of hours. For more information on Group B strep, see page 103.

Also, once the bag of waters breaks, the pregnant person should take precautions to prevent bacteria from entering the uterus, as this might increase the chance of infection. Put nothing in the vagina—no tampons; no penetrative intercourse; no checking the cervix with fingers. Taking a tub bath is okay and will not increase the chance of infection, provided the tub is clean.

Until the laboring person is clearly in active labor, the caregiver and nurses should be very cautious about doing vaginal exams to assess the cervix for dilation. Such exams tend to push bacteria through the cervix into the uterus and increase the chances of infection. Even if you're curious about dilation, do not ask for a vaginal exam. You should also question the nurse or caregiver who wants to do one. Collecting fluid for testing is an exception to this rule; because the speculum and swab do not enter the cervix, this procedure poses little risk of infection.

If precautions are followed and the pregnant person does not carry Group B streptococcus, it is probably safely to wait for labor to begin spontaneously. The caregiver probably won't think it necessary to induce labor, sometimes for a day or more. Most caregivers have a policy regarding management of ruptured membranes (broken bag of waters); some induce labor within hours after the baq breaks; others wait. It is wise to ask about this policy ahead of time. If the pregnant person is at low risk for infection (for example, having tested negative for Group B strep and has had no vaginal exams), it is reasonable to ask to delay induction for a day or more.

> **CAUTION:** On very rare occasions, when the bag of waters breaks with a gush of fluid, the baby's umbilical cord slips below the baby or out of the uterus as the water escapes. This is called prolapsed cord and is a **true emergency** (see "Prolapsed Cord," page 131).

"FALSE" LABOR, OR PRELABOR

Frequently, pregnant people have contractions that are quite strong and frequent, but they are *nonprogressing*—that is, the pattern of contractions remains the same. The contractions do not become longer, stronger, or closer together over time. When examined, these people may be told they are in "false" labor, which means the cervix is not yet opening (dilating). The term *prelabor* is much more appropriate because there is nothing "false" about these contractions, and they accomplish changes that allow "true" labor (that is, dilation) to occur. Prelabor contractions are also called Braxton Hicks contractions. Many people who are examined in prelabor and told it is not labor feel discouraged and embarrassed at the error and may lose faith in their ability to recognize labor, or they may feel distressed and confused if admitted to the hospital. The support the pregnant person receives from you or a doula in these circumstances is critical to their ability to cope with "true" progressing labor later. Here is how you can help:

- Most importantly, point out that "false" labor does not mean what they are experiencing is not real. All it means is the cervix has not yet begun to open. Refer to the contractions as "prelabor" instead.
- Remind the pregnant person that opening (dilation) of the cervix beyond about 2 centimeters is one of the last things to happen, after the cervix has moved into position, ripened, and effaced. The fact that the cervix is not yet opening does not mean there is no progress.
- If the pregnant parent becomes discouraged with a prolonged period of nonprogressing contractions, remind them of the six ways that labor progresses (see "Labor Progresses in Six Ways," page 24).

- Ask the caregiver who examines the pregnant parent whether the cervix has moved forward, softened further, or thinned more. Sometimes, the caregiver is so focused on the opening of the cervix (dilation), these other important signs of progress are not mentioned.
- If the laboring person does not want to go home, you might walk around outside the hospital or hang out in the cafeteria or lobby to see if the contractions progress further. If they don't change, you might be more comfortable at home.

See "Prelabor," page 29, and "The Slow-to-Start Labor," page 92, for strategies to help the laboring person cope with these early contractions. You can be sure that if the laboring person has either of the Positive Signs of labor listed in the table on page 68, the cervix is opening. The pregnant person cannot be in "false" labor if, over a period of time, the contractions have become longer, stronger, *and* closer together or at least two of those three things occur (see "Timing Contractions," page 26).

LABOR PROGRESSES IN SIX WAYS

A laboring person makes progress toward birth in the following ways. Note that significant dilation does not take place until step 4. The first three steps usually occur simultaneously and gradually over the last weeks of pregnancy and into early labor.

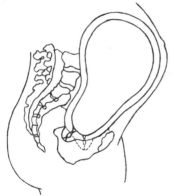

The cervix moves from the posterior to the anterior position late in pregnancy or early in labor.

1. **The cervix softens (ripens).** While still thick, the cervix, through the action of hormones and prostaglandins, softens and becomes more pliable.
2. **The position of the cervix changes.** The cervix points toward the pregnant parent's back during most of pregnancy and then gradually moves forward. The position of the cervix is assessed by a vaginal exam and is described as posterior (pointing toward the back), midline, or anterior (pointing toward the front).

3. **The cervix thins and shortens (effaces).** Usually about 1½ inches (3.5 cm) long, the cervix gradually shortens and becomes paper-thin. The amount of thinning (effacement) is measured in two ways:

   Percentages: Zero percent means no thinning or shortening has occurred; 50 percent means the cervix is about half its former thickness; 100 percent means it is paper-thin.

Centimeters of length: One and one-half inches (3.5 cm) is the same as 0 percent effaced; ¾ inch (2 cm) long is the same as 50 percent effaced; and less than ½ inch (1 cm) long means 80 to 90 percent effaced. Do not confuse centimeters of cervical length with centimeters of cervical dilation!

4. **The cervix opens (dilates).** The opening (dilation) of the cervix is also measured in centimeters. The measurement is estimated by the caregiver who inserts two fingers through the cervix, spreads the fingers to the edges of the cervix, and estimates how far apart (in centimeters) the fingers are—it is not an exact science. Dilation usually occurs with progressing contractions—after the cervix has undergone the changes just described—but it is common for the cervix to dilate 1 to 3 centimeters before the pregnant person has Positive Signs of labor. The cervix must open to approximately 10 centimeters in diameter to allow the baby through.

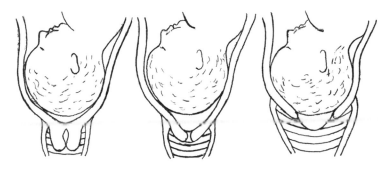

A cervix that has not effaced or dilated and is 3–4 cm (1 to 1½ inches) long

A cervix that is 75 percent effaced (about 1 cm long [½ inch] and 1 cm (½ inch) dilated

A cervix that is 100 percent effaced (or paper-thin) and 4 cm (1½ inches) dilated; the bag of waters is bulging

5. **The baby's chin tucks onto the chest (called flexion) and the head rotates.** The rotation makes it easier for the baby to pass through the birth canal. (Sometimes, especially if the head is large, it must "mold" before it can rotate. This means the head changes shape, becoming longer and thinner. Molding is normal, although some babies' heads look somewhat misshapen for a day or two following birth, after which they return to a round shape.) The most favorable position for birth is usually the OA (occiput anterior) position; see page 96 for information on other positions.

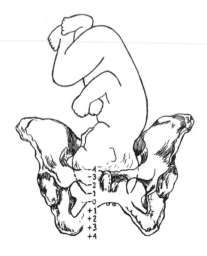

Station—a measure of the baby's descent

6. The baby descends. The head continues to mold as necessary to fit and descends through the cervix, the pelvis, and the vagina to the outside. The descent is described in terms of "station," which tells how far above or below the pregnant person's midpelvis the baby's head is (or buttocks or feet, in the case of a breech presentation); is measured in centimeters; and ranges from minus 4 to plus 4. A "zero station" means the baby's head is right at midpelvis. Minus 1, 2, 3, or 4 means the head is that number of centimeters above midpelvis. The greater the "plus" number, the closer the baby's head is to the outside and to being born.

Some descent usually takes place before labor begins, especially for first-time labors. When the baby "drops," it settles into the pelvis to about minus 2 or minus 1. Most of the descent occurs late in labor.

Steps 4 through 6 (dilation beyond 2 to 3 centimeters, rotation, and descent) cannot take place until the first three steps are well under way. In other words, a firm, thick, or posterior cervix won't open. It simply is not ready. And a baby won't rotate and descend significantly until the cervix is open. For many laboring people, the first three steps take place imperceptibly and gradually in late pregnancy. For others, they take place in a few days, with strong or even painful nonprogressing contractions, referred to as "prelabor" contractions (see page 23).

TIMING CONTRACTIONS

In early labor, one of the important jobs of the birth partner is to time contractions. Changes in the length, strength, and frequency of contractions are the all-important hallmarks of true progressing labor, so it is a good idea for you to know how to time them correctly and keep a written record. When you call the caregiver, you will have accurate and concrete information to provide.

The easiest way to time contractions is with smartphone with an application for timing contractions. There are many available. Search the app store for "contraction timer," or something similar, or see our Recommended Resources on page 190. The laboring person indicates the beginning and end of the contractions and one of you taps the screen or presses a key. The smartphone keeps track of duration and frequency. You can enter other information such as that shown in the "Comments" column in the table on page 189. Keep track of five or six in a row to record the contraction pattern. Then, you may wait until the contraction pattern seems to have changed. Time five or six more contractions and resume timing when the contractions are clearly stronger. Continue this until it is time to call the hospital.

A note of caution: Many apps provide an "average duration" and "average frequency." Often, this can give the impression the contractions are closer together than they actually are and may cause you to leave for the hospital too soon.

It's important to look for the one key indicator: contractions that have become *longer, stronger, and closer together (or at least two of these criteria) over time.* Once these criteria have been met and the pattern reaches 4-1-1 or 5-1-1 (see page 33), it is time to go to the place of birth.

When you call the caregiver or the hospital's labor floor, have the information near you and be prepared to report what you recorded. (Make sure you know whom to call. Some caregivers prefer you call them directly; others want you to call the hospital's labor-and-delivery area and talk to a nurse.)

Note: When timing contractions and considering the interval, or how far apart the contractions are, it is important to count from the *start* of one contraction to the *start* of the next. Don't fall into the trap of timing from the end of one to the start of the next, as you will go to your place of birth or call your birth team too soon!

See page 33 for the discussion "When Do You Go to the Hospital or Settle in for a Home Birth?"

Now that you know how to tell when labor is underway, you're ready to read the next chapter about what happens during labor.

CHAPTER 3

Moving Through the Stages of Labor

Labor and birth rate among the most intense of all normal human experiences because they are so demanding— physically, emotionally, and mentally. This is true not only for the person in labor, but also for those who love and care for that person. Labor is unpredictable, empowering, and fulfilling—and it comes with a great prize at the end!

The most predictable thing about childbirth is its total unpredictability. A pregnant person does not know when labor will begin, how long it will take, or how painful it will be, or whether problems will arise that may require medical treatment. They do not know whether or how it might be similar or different from their mother's labors or the labors of other people. They cannot even be sure to get a good night's sleep beforehand! And they cannot predict what the postpartum course will be like.

This unpredictability of childbirth may be a source of frustration or anxiety for both of you as you learn what to expect and how to help. Partners in our childbirth classes often ask questions such as these:

- Once the cervix has begun to ripen, how long does it usually take before labor starts?
- After contractions begin, how many hours before we should go to the hospital?
- How long is the pushing stage?
- When should I take time off from work?
- How bad will the pain get?
- When do babies sleep through the night?
- How long do people breastfeed?

Questions like these usually receive evasive answers: "It may be hours or days. You can be sure it is a sign they are moving in the right direction." "It varies." "We can't be sure." "People experience things differently." "It's hard to say."

Birth partners want to know exactly what to prepare for, but it is simply not possible to answer these questions precisely. Variations are inherent in childbirth because each human being and each labor is unique. The key is to accept the unpredictability and pace yourselves while the labor process unfolds.

There is good news, however. Despite all the uncertainties, there are some things you can count on. This chapter gives you a broad idea of what you can expect from this mysterious process. You will learn the wide range of normal possibilities and how you can be truly helpful. The emotions experienced by laboring people constitute a large part of the discussion, along with the emotional responses you may have. Here, you'll find practical and useful suggestions to help with the challenging task of providing the laboring person emotional support as well as physical comfort.

The following terms describe what happens during labor and how the laboring person may respond:

- Prelabor refers to the time before labor actually begins, when the pregnant person experiences nonprogressing contractions (see below) and the cervix is changing, but not yet dilating. The contractions may come and go for a period of hours to days.
- The first stage of labor (often simply called labor) is the dilation stage, during which the cervix dilates completely—to about 10 centimeters in diameter. The contractions progress over time, becoming longer, stronger, and/or closer together.
- The second stage is the pushing and birthing stage, during which the baby is born.
- The third stage is the placental stage, during which the placenta, or afterbirth, is born.
- The fourth stage is the recovery and bonding stage during which the birthing parent and baby get to know each other and the first feedings occur.

See the illustrations of each stage and phase of labor on page 43.

The dilation (first) and birthing (second) stages are further divided (four phases in the first stage and three in the second). With every new phase, labor changes its rhythm, and the laboring person must make an emotional adjustment. This chapter describes each stage and phase and includes suggestions for how you and a doula can help the laboring person cope.

PRELABOR

Prelabor is the phase that precedes actual labor. See chapter 2 for a detailed discussion of prelabor. This is the time when you and the laboring person are likely to be on your own or with an anxious relative or friend. If you understand what is happening and how to help, you have a better chance of getting to the hospital or birth center or gathering the birth team for a home birth at the appropriate time—neither too early nor too late.

Getting to the hospital too early means either that the pregnant person will be sent home or that medical interventions to start labor may be performed essentially out of impatience ("They're here; let's get labor going."). Medical interventions don't always succeed, and they tend to pile up—one intervention leading to another. If you can avoid this cascade of interventions by going to the hospital at the proper time, the pregnant person will have a better chance of a normal delivery. In fact, the American College of Obstetricians and Gynecologists, which sets guidelines for maternity care, strongly recommends NOT being admitted to the hospital too early as a way to avoid unnecessary medical treatment, including cesarean delivery. We want to help you feel confident in staying home until the right time. .

Before going on, we should mention that a small percentage of pregnant parents, first-time and not, never experience much of what we have just described. They skip the preliminaries and begin having progressing contractions as soon as they are aware they are having contractions. Sometimes, when they look back, they realize that the restless night's sleep or the crampy, soft bowel movements must have been prelabor. Others have no warm-up. They plunge immediately into labor.

WHAT IS PRELABOR LIKE FOR THE PREGNANT PERSON HAVING A SECOND OR SUBSEQUENT CHILD?

Prelabor is often different for the experienced parent. Strong contractions may continue for a while, especially at night, even progressing enough to convince them they are in labor, but then subside by morning and resume the next night. This "on-again-off-again" contraction pattern is not unusual for an experienced pregnant person. They may be 3 or 4 centimeters dilated but not yet be in labor! While such a pattern can be frustrating, think of it this way: "You're dilating, and you aren't even in labor!" Once labor actually gets going, it is usually faster than the first, though there are exceptions.

As you can see, prelabor can be a confusing time for the pregnant person, birth partner, and even the caregiver. You may find it difficult to distinguish between this tuning up and the "real thing." Then, without warning, and perhaps without either of you recognizing it, prelabor contractions become the "real thing"—getting longer, stronger, and/or closer together. The cervix begins to dilate.

HOW LONG DOES PRELABOR LAST?

Prelabor may last from a few hours to many hours, or it may come and go over several days.

WHAT THE CAREGIVER DOES

Depending on your report, the caregiver may suggest that the laboring person wait at home, come into the office for a progress check, or go straight to the hospital or birth center. In addition, the caregiver may do any of the following:

- Come to your home to check the laboring person, if a home birth is planned. Depending on the midwife's findings, they may leave or stay.
- Offer advice and encouragement to help handle this frustrating phase.
- Suggest a warm bath or medication for rest or to slow contractions if prelabor has been going on for a long time.
- Try to speed labor with medications or by breaking the bag of waters (see "Induction or Augmentation of Labor," page 114).

HOW YOU CAN HELP

Assist the laboring person with prelabor in these ways:

- Realize that a long prelabor, though challenging, is not a medical problem in itself. Therefore, it is mostly up to the two of you to handle it, perhaps with the help of a doula, friends, or family members.

- Recognize prelabor for what it is. Help the laboring person determine whether the contractions are progressing by timing them occasionally. If they are not progressing, point out that labor will feel clearly different from what is currently happening (see "Timing Contractions," page 26; "Signs of Labor," page 21; and "'False' Labor, or Prelabor," page 29).
- If you have a doula, call them to discuss ways you can help the laboring person and when they should come. If you are getting tired or discouraged, the doula might come and help so you can get some rest.
- Check with the caregiver for advice and reassurance and possibly to arrange an examination.
- Encourage the laboring person to eat when hungry and drink when thirsty.
- Do projects or activities together to help get your minds off the contractions. You might give a massage, or the two of you might prepare food, play games, go for a walk, visit with friends, or read a book aloud to each other. If the laboring person likes to color or do crafts, have the necessary materials on hand.
- Consult "The Slow-to-Start Labor," page 92, for specific coping techniques if prelabor continues for a long time.

THE DILATION, FIRST, STAGE

Dilation, or the opening of the cervix, occurs in the first stage of labor. Dilation begins about when the prelabor contractions change from their nonprogressing pattern to becoming longer, stronger, and closer together (or at least two of those three). The first stage ends when the cervix has dilated completely (to approximately 10 centimeters). The dilation stage can proceed very quickly, unevenly, or slowly. It has distinct phases: the latent phase (also called early labor), the active phase (or active labor), and the transition phase (or just transition; see illustrations, page 43).

The change from prelabor to the dilation stage may be gradual, so don't expect that either of you will know the moment the cervix begins to open.

In a "textbook" labor, the contractions gradually and steadily increase in intensity and duration and come closer together. Early contractions may last from 30 to 40 seconds and come anywhere from 5 to 20 minutes apart. Although there are exceptions, these early contractions are usually painless. As they progress in length, frequency, and duration, they become more intense and painful. By the time the cervix opens to 8 or 9 centimeters, the contractions may last 90 seconds or more, feel very intense (almost surely very painful), and come every 2 to 4 minutes. The pain of labor usually reaches its maximum by 7 or 8 centimeters. Second-stage contractions are different and may not be painful or may be painful in a different way (see pages 45–48).

HOW LONG DOES THE DILATION STAGE LAST?

The dilation stage lasts from 2 to 24 hours, although for first-time labors, it rarely lasts fewer than 4 hours.

You cannot know in advance how long dilation will take, but the way labor starts may give you some clues. If the labor starts right off with contractions that seem very long or very painful and close together, you may wonder whether these are the relatively easy ones you've been expecting. You must trust the laboring person's perceptions and yours. Their labor might be one of those uncommon, very fast ones. Call the caregiver or the hospital, give an accurate idea of what is happening, and get the caregiver's or nurse's advice. Try not to worry; a very fast labor usually means everything is normal (almost too normal!). Turn immediately to chapter 5, for a discussion of the very rapid labor.

In a slow labor, contractions continue as quite manageable and progress very gradually over a long period of time. This can lead to discouragement, fatigue, and worry. You'll both need to pace yourselves through an extra-long labor (see "Arrest of Active Labor [Dystocia]," page 129).

WHEN TO CALL THE CAREGIVER OR HOSPITAL?

Make sure you have the correct numbers to call (see chapter 1) and call under any of the following circumstances:

- Signs of labor before 37 weeks—a premature labor (see "Signs of Labor," page 21)
- Leaking or a gush of fluid from the vagina (see "If the Bag of Waters Breaks Before Labor Begins," page 22)
- Contractions clearly becoming longer, stronger, and closer together (see "Signs of Labor," page 21; "The 4-1-1 or 5-1-1 Rule," page 33; and "Timing Contractions," page 26)
- You or the laboring person has questions or concerns
- If the pregnant parent has given birth before, call the caregiver or hospital when the contractions are progressing and the pregnant person thinks or knows labor has started. A second (or later) labor is usually faster than a first one.

Early Labor

This first phase of the dilation stage lasts until the cervix is dilated to 5 or 6 centimeters. Medical professionals call this the *latent phase* of the first stage.

The big difference between prelabor and early labor is that during early labor, the cervix begins to open gradually. For the laboring person, birth partner, and doula, this shift to early labor is signaled by clearly progressing contractions. The caregiver uses vaginal exams as necessary to determine changes in the cervix during this phase.

HOW LONG DOES EARLY LABOR LAST?

Typically, early labor takes from two-thirds to three-quarters of the total time of the dilation stage. In other words, it could take from a few hours to 20 hours or so for a person in labor to reach 5 or 6 centimeters of dilation. The length of early labor depends largely on the state of the cervix, the position and station of the baby within the pelvis at the time labor begins, and the strength of the contractions. Chances for more rapid progress are increased if the following conditions exist:

- The cervix has moved forward and is very soft and thin (see page 24).
- The contractions are intense and close together.
- The baby is in the occiput anterior (OA) position, with head down, chin on chest, and the back of the head toward the pregnant person's front (see page 96). You and

the pregnant person really can't tell the position of the baby; it is also difficult for the caregiver to tell.

- The baby's head has begun to move down into the pelvis.

These favorable conditions increase the likelihood of an average or shorter-than-average early labor. Under any other conditions, early labor is likely to take longer than the rest of labor. Labor is not a race against time, however. A normal early labor can last from a few hours to many hours.

WHAT THE CAREGIVER OR LABOR-AND-DELIVERY STAFF DO

During early labor, the caregiver or hospital staff can help in the following ways.

- Giving advice over the telephone; when you call, be prepared to provide the information recorded on the Early Labor Record (see page 189).

THE 4-1-1 OR 5-1-1 RULE

Before going to the hospital or birth center, wait until the contractions have been 4 to 5 minutes apart and 1 minute long for at least 1 hour. Whether you use 4-1-1 or 5-1-1 depends on the caregiver's preferences, the laboring person's preference, whether this is a first or subsequent labor, how far you are from the hospital or birth center, and whether there is considered high risk of complications.

- Helping the laboring person decide when to go to the hospital. If it is not yet time to go, they may advise some things to do until it is time.
- Advising when to go to the caregiver's office or hospital for assessment of the contractions and, perhaps, a vaginal exam for an idea of how dilation is progressing.

WHEN DO YOU GO TO THE HOSPITAL?

Under most circumstances, the first-time laboring parent should go to the hospital or birth center or settle in for a home birth when they have had 10 to 15 consecutive contractions that:

- Last at least 1 minute
- Are 4 to 5 minutes apart (or closer)
- Are strong enough they cannot be distracted from them
- Are strong enough they must use a breathing, relaxation, or attention- focusing ritual (see page 55) to get through them

Usually, it takes about an hour to time the contractions and determine whether they fit this pattern. If they are less than 4 minutes apart and advancing quickly, however, do not wait an hour before going to the hospital or birth center.

Sometimes, there are reasons for going to the hospital earlier than described here. For example:

- The pregnant person lives a long distance from the hospital.
- There are medical problems that require early admission. The caregiver will advise whether these problems exist.

- The pregnant person has given birth before (especially if the first labor was very rapid) and recognizes that labor has started. A second (or later) labor usually goes faster than the first one.
- They are anxious and really want to be at the hospital or birth center. Note: If the plan is to give birth in an out-of-hospital birth center, do not go there without calling the midwife to set a time to meet at the birth center. The facility may be locked and unstaffed, especially at night.

Because early labor can take a long time, it is often a good idea to spend the time relaxing together or with friends until the contractions fit the pattern described here. It is usually best not to arrive at the hospital (or call the caregiver to the home) too early because:

- The laboring person may feel "performance anxiety"—pressure to start producing some good contractions. They may feel watched by the caregiver or nurse, who seems to be waiting for something to happen, and may feel something is wrong because labor is so slow.
- The laboring person may become unnecessarily preoccupied with the contractions and the apparent lack of progress, and this may make labor seem longer or more difficult than it is.
- The laboring person may become bored, anxious, or discouraged.
- The staff may offer or suggest medical interventions to speed up this normally slow part of labor. You and the laboring person should ask the key questions (see page 101) before considering these interventions. They all carry some risks, including the possibility they will not succeed and then other interventions may be required. Without a medical need, these interventions may carry more risk than benefit.

Sometimes, the caregiver will recommend that you and the laboring person leave the hospital or birth center and come back later. For a home birth, everyone except you may have to leave for a while. Although discouraging, this measure allows the labor to settle into its own pattern and takes pressure off the laboring person.

HOW YOU CAN HELP

Your role now is very similar to the role you played during prelabor. Remain close by; supply the laboring person with food and drink; time five or six contractions, when the pattern seems to change; and help the laboring person pass the time with pleasant and distracting activities (see "The Slow-to-Start Labor," page 92).

At some point, the labor pattern will intensify and the laboring person will become preoccupied with the contractions, no longer able to walk or talk through them without pausing; the contractions "stop them in their tracks." From this point on, it is not appropriate to leave or to distract them. Instead, do the following:

- Give the laboring person your undivided attention throughout every contraction. Stop what you are doing and stop talking so you can focus. Do not ask questions during contractions.

- Watch during the contractions and, if you notice tension, help the laboring person relax their entire body during each one (see "Relaxation," page 58).
- Suggest using the planned ritual ("relax, breathe, and focus")—slow, rhythmic breathing while focusing on something pleasant or positive, such as letting go of tension with each exhale (see page 61).
- Encourage slow, rhythmic breathing through comforting touch and verbal encouragement during each contraction ("That's good. . . . Just like that.") and helpful comments when the contraction is over ("You relaxed very well that time," or "I noticed you tensed your shoulders with that contraction; with the next one, focus on keeping your shoulders relaxed.").
- Help decide when to call the caregiver.
- If you have hired one, but not yet called your doula, call now, either to alert them that you expect to need them soon or to ask them to join you.
  What does a doula do? Beginning with your phone call, the doula will probably:
- Ask what's happening. Tell the doula about the signs of labor, the contraction pattern, and how you both feel and are coping.
- Ask to speak to the laboring person and assess their distractibility.
- Listen to the laboring person through a contraction to get an idea of how they are coping (does the breathing or moaning sound relaxed or tense?) and to encourage them in their planned ritual, perhaps by breathing audibly with them through the contraction. This will help the laboring person relax and breathe rhythmically.
- Ask the laboring person the all-important question: "What was going through your mind during that contraction?" As the doula listens to the laboring person's response, they assess whether the laboring person is positive and coping well or feeling distressed.
- Be sure you and the laboring person know if the doula can or will come to your home in early labor. Sometimes, it is not realistic due to distance; some doulas have a policy of joining you at the hospital or birth center. Be sure you know in advance.

If the laboring person is coping well and you do not indicate otherwise, the doula will probably decide not to come yet, but will remind you of things to do and make a plan for staying in touch.

If the laboring person is distressed or asks the doula to come, the doula may suggest some coping strategies to try until they arrive and will hurry to join you. The doula should tell you when and where they'll arrive—at your home, the hospital, or the birth center.

When the doula joins you, they will:

- Wash their hands, and, if you are at the hospital or birth center, meet the staff
- Assess the laboring person's needs and your feelings
- Assist as appropriate, keeping in mind your planned support role, which you, the laboring person, and the doula discussed in a previous meeting
- Sit quietly through a contraction or two to observe the two of you working together so their role will fit with what you are doing

- Help you determine when to go to the hospital or birth center, if you are still at home Early labor eventually evolves into a more intense pattern of progressing contractions.

Getting into Active Labor (3 to 6 Centimeters Dilation)

You need to know that during the time from 3 to 6 centimeters an emotional shift takes place in many laboring people, and the support they need from their partner and doula changes. We call this period the "3 to 6 phase," or "getting into active labor." This is also likely to be when contractions reach the point when you should go to the hospital or birth center or that your home birth midwife should be called (see 4-1-1 or 5-1-1, pages 33).

It is not unusual for the laboring person to have a cervical exam and be told the cervix has not dilated much. This is discouraging. The explanation is that even though the contractions have increased in intensity and duration, the cervix may not yet be ready to dilate. It may require time to ripen, thin, or move forward enough to begin dilating (see pages 24–26). We sometimes say "3 to 6" is the time when the laboring person turns the corner into active labor. Your help with comfort measures (see chapter 4), along with guidance and reassurance from a doula or other knowledgeable person, help the laboring person understand what is happening and manage the more intense contractions. And, if necessary, pain medications are available in the hospital (see chapter 8). Note that "3 to 6" may take 2 to 4 hours or possibly more.

HOW WILL THE LABORING PERSON FEEL?

We sometimes refer to this phase as the "moment of truth," when the laboring person realizes, in a new and powerful way, they cannot control this labor. Earlier optimism may give way to a temporary loss of confidence or a struggle to remain "in control." They may worry that labor is too difficult or weep from discouragement and a sense of a long way to go. They may want pain medications, even if that wasn't the original plan. As they struggle with the lack of control, the laboring person comes to realize they can't do it with will or determination alone and may give up trying to control it. One woman said, "I can't do this; I'm done." As she stopped "thinking her way through the contractions," things changed for the better. This time is often a turning point. If the laboring person doesn't feel judged and feels emotionally "safe," they are likely to become more instinctual and find their "spontaneous ritual"—their own way to cope during the contractions (see pages 55–58).

WHAT THE CAREGIVER OR LABOR-AND-DELIVERY STAFF DO

If the laboring person has not already been admitted to the hospital or birth center, they will be now. If a home birth is planned, the midwife will try to get there at this time.

HOW YOU CAN HELP

Recognize the change in mood; don't try to distract the laboring person—no jokes or games anymore. Don't minimize their worries. Stay calm, use a soothing "labor voice," and murmur soothing, encouraging words. Help them maintain a rhythm. Use comfort measures (slow dancing, massage, visualizations, rhythmic breathing, and moaning). Acknowledge that this is difficult, but don't give up. Offer support using the 3 Rs (relaxation, rhythm, and ritual) through the contractions (page 55). Support their original preferences regarding the use of pain medications. If the original plan was to use pain medications, this might be a good time to get them. If the plan was to minimize or postpone medications, encourage the laboring person to continue. Try a change in ritual for a few contractions: Walk, use light breathing (see pages 63–64), try a massage (see pages 80–85), or the Take-Charge routine (see pages 86–88). A doula can advise and help with comfort techniques and explanations of what is happening and what to expect. The good news is that once the laboring person gets through this phase, they will have found a way to cope, and the contractions will likely be more manageable.

Active Labor

The active phase of labor begins when the cervix is thin and soft and contractions are closer and stronger. At this point, the cervix has dilated to about 6 centimeters and now begins to dilate faster (although in some labors the cervix is ready to dilate quickly before 6 centimeters). Active labor lasts until cervical dilation reaches about 8 centimeters.

During active labor, contractions intensify, still lasting more than 1 minute and coming every 3 to 4 minutes. The contractions are usually very intense, and most laboring people describe them as very painful, but manageable.

It is important to recognize the positive meanings of active labor. As demanding as the contractions are, they mean labor is progressing well and the laboring body is doing exactly what it needs to do. The pain is not a danger sign; rather, it is a side effect of the strong contractions, the pressure in the uterus, and the stretching of the cervix that will bring the baby into the world. It is possible for many laboring people to cope with these intense contractions when they have had good support through the "3 to 6" phase; that is, they know ways to reduce the pain and stay relaxed; have continuous feedback from positive partners; and experience a reasonably normal labor pattern.

HOW LONG DOES ACTIVE LABOR LAST?

Normally, active labor is much shorter than early labor and the "3 to 6" phase. For first-time laboring people, active labor usually ranges from 3 to 7 hours. It is usually much faster for those who have had babies before—from 20 minutes to 3 hours.

WHAT THE LABORING PERSON FEELS

The person in labor must make an emotional adjustment to the changing rhythm and sensations of labor, becoming focused on coping with the more frequent and intense contractions, and may not even realize the pace of dilation is picking up or will soon. Response to the changing rhythm of labor may include:

- Feeling tired and discouraged as they realize the tough part is just beginning, or they may have found a ritual and be very focused during each contraction. With support and encouragement, their mood will likely turn to acceptance, and they will discover their own way to handle the contractions.
- Extraneous conversation becomes annoying. The laboring person may feel very alone if you and others do not recognize this change and continue trying to distract or, worse, ignore them and talk to one another.

- When the laboring person lets their body take over, they become serious and focused on the contractions. They devote all attention to maintaining a rhythmic ritual—releasing tension, breathing, moving, or moaning during contractions. When a contraction ends, conversation, if any, is likely to consist of reviewing it with you and talking about what to do for the next one.
- With your understanding and good support, the laboring person will be able to get past this crisis, let go of the need to be in control, and work with, not against, the contractions, by letting the body take over. We call these unplanned coping techniques spontaneous rituals.

At this time, the laboring person benefits from a quiet room, freedom to move around in and out of bed, and as little disturbance or interruption as possible. They may want to be held or stroked or, conversely, not touched at all. This is when laboring people become more instinctual, more focused, and less verbal. You might think when labor is steadily advancing, people would find it more and more difficult to cope. But this is not the case when laboring people feel well supported. They actually find it easier to cope once they release the need to be in control because they let their bodies take over, become more instinctual in their behavior, and discover what works for them.

WHAT THE CAREGIVER DOES

In a hospital birth, generally, the doctor isn't in the birth room very much during active labor but is available nearby or by telephone. A nurse provides most of the direct clinical care, following the doctor's orders. If the caregiver is a midwife, they are likely to provide more care than a doctor, but the nurse is a major figure in carrying out the midwife's orders.

As labor advances, the midwife or nurse becomes more actively involved. Now that progress is faster and the contractions are more intense, closer surveillance is needed. The nurse or midwife checks the laboring person's:

- Blood pressure, pulse, and temperature
- Fluid intake and urine output
- Length, intensity, and frequency of contractions
- Dilation of the cervix

In addition, the nurse or midwife also checks the baby's heart rate and position and station (see page 26).

Routines vary, depending on the management style of the caregiver. Some obstetricians rely heavily on routine interventions and medical technology. For example, breaking the bag of waters, restricting the laboring person to bed, giving intravenous (IV) fluids, using electronic fetal monitoring to continuously check the fetus and the contractions, giving the laboring person medications to speed the labor and relieve pain, performing an episiotomy (a surgical incision to enlarge the vaginal opening just before birth), and, if the birth is taking too long and progressing too slowly, use forceps, a vacuum extractor, or cesarean surgery to deliver the baby.

Other obstetricians and most midwives and family doctors rely on simpler methods. They might encourage a healthy person at low risk for complications to drink liquids and move around. They might listen to the fetal heartbeat with a handheld Doppler ultrasound device or use the electronic fetal monitor off and on through the labor rather than continuously. They might suggest comfort measures (see chapter 4) to relieve pain before offering an epidural or other drugs.

Midwives and family doctors tend to intervene less than most obstetricians, partly because of training, but also because midwives and family doctors are more likely to care for people with healthy pregnancies and few risks of medical problems in labor. Obstetricians care for people at both low and high risk for problems, and many tend to use procedures for all patients that are really only needed for high-risk pregnancies. See chapter 6 for information about commonly used tests and procedures and also for key questions to ask and alternatives to consider.

The nurse or caregiver may offer helpful advice and reassurance. Having someone there with expertise and experience—someone you both trust—can be immensely reassuring. Don't hesitate to ask for help or advice if you feel uncertain about the labor or about how you can help the person in labor.

HOW YOU CAN HELP
Your role during active labor is very important. How you respond to the laboring person's needs determines, to a large extent, how well they cope and will feel later about the birth experience. Here are some guidelines for helping during this phase:

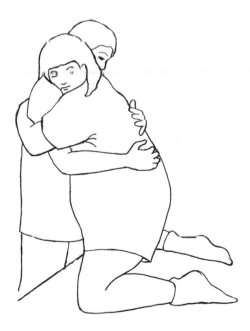

- Make sure staff are aware of the birth plan, especially regarding to preferences for pain medications and other interventions. See chapter 1, and chapter 8.
- Follow the laboring person's lead. Take your cues from them; match their mood. If serious or quiet, you be serious or quiet. Don't try to jolly them out of this mood or distract them at this time. Labor takes almost all their attention, and they need you physically and emotionally.
- Acknowledge feelings. If the laboring person says, "I can't do this," you might reply, "This is rough. Let me help you more. Keep your rhythm."
- Offer liquid to drink after each contraction or two. Don't disturb the laboring person by asking what they would like to drink; just hold the beverage where it can be seen. It will be taken if wanted, ignored if not, or a different beverage may be requested. Don't pressure them to drink more, unless the caregiver is concerned about fluid intake. Otherwise, they should drink when thirsty.
- Give the laboring person your undivided attention throughout every contraction, even when their eyes are closed and you think it's not needed. Do not ask questions during contractions as they may interrupt or disturb the coping ritual. Do not chat with others in the room and discourage others from engaging in nonessential or loud conversation. Such talk could make the laboring person feel very alone and ignored, even when coping well.
- Help with comfort measures. Hold the laboring person and slow dance; rub their shoulders or press on their back; walk with them; stay beside the shower or bathtub or get in, too, (bring a swimsuit for this purpose). For more suggestions, see chapter 4.
- Remember, rhythm is everything. Rhythm is key to coping in the dilation stage. If there is rhythm in whatever the laboring person does during contractions (moaning, swaying, tapping, rocking, chanting, even silent self-talk) or whatever they want you to do (holding them, stroking them, swaying together, talking, nodding your head, moaning together), they are coping. Being "in their rhythm" means matching or mirroring their rhythm with your words, movements, or touch. It is a way to share the experience closely and provide strong appropriate guidance.

If the laboring person loses rhythm and tenses, grimaces, writhes, clutches, or cries out, they need your help (or the doula's or nurse's) to regain the rhythm they had or to find a new one. If you have been in their rhythm, it's much easier to help them get it back. At times, you might help by making eye contact or by rhythmically talking, stroking, or swaying along with laboring person (see "The Take-Charge Routine," page 86).

Do give rhythm top priority to keep the laboring person from feeling overwhelmed and to help maintain a sense of mastery during this challenging part of labor. Let them stick with the same rhythmic ritual as long as it helps. Don't be afraid to suggest something new, though, if the laboring person loses the rhythm and has real trouble getting back to it. Labor sometimes becomes so stressful that they will need to follow someone else's lead. They will let you know when it's time to return to the previous ritual.

Transition

The transition phase is another turning point in labor—from the dilation to the birthing stage. In this phase, the laboring person's body seems to be partly in the dilation (first) stage and partly in the birthing (second) stage.

During transition, the cervix dilates the last 1 to 2 centimeters; (from about 8 or 9 centimeters to about 10) and the baby begins to descend. The head moves from within the uterus through the cervix and down into the vagina (see illustrations, page 43). Contractions have reached maximum intensity, each lasting 1 to 2 minutes and occurring very close together.

Sometimes, a "lip" of cervix delays the last bit of dilation. A "lip" occurs when a part of the cervix remains thick after most of the cervix has completely dilated. This may be caused by the position of the baby's head, which may press unevenly against the cervix. Several contractions or more may be needed to draw the cervix out of the way so the baby's head can come through. Changing the laboring person's position, using hands and knees, open knee–chest, or lunging may help reduce the lip. (See also chapter 4.)

The uterus may begin its expulsive action even before the cervix is completely dilated. We call this the "urge to push." It causes the laboring person to catch their breath, grunt, or hold their breath and strain; this is what is meant by the terms *pushing* and *bearing down*.

The urge to push is an involuntary reflex; the laboring person does not make it happen and cannot prevent it from happening. Yet, if the cervix is not completely dilated, they may begin bearing down very slightly. We call this "grunt-pushing." This may happen instinctively or the nurse or caregiver may instruct the laboring person to strain just enough to satisfy the urge. Pushing very hard before the cervix is dilated could cause the cervix to swell and the labor to slow (see "Avoiding Forceful Pushing," page 64).

HOW LONG DOES TRANSITION LAST?

The transition usually takes between 5 to 30 contractions or from 15 minutes to a couple hours. If the cervix has a lip or the baby's head is not well positioned (or both), the transition phase will likely take longer.

WHAT THE CAREGIVER DOES

During the transition phase, a nurse or a midwife is in almost constant attendance. The doctor is not necessarily with the laboring person, although when informed that delivery is very close, the doctor soon comes.

The nurse or the midwife may do any or all of the following:

- Check the cervix to confirm the progress of labor
- Ask the laboring person not to push or to push only gently, with little grunts, if the cervix is not fully opened
- Reassure the laboring person that all is right and labor is moving rapidly
- Help you in your birth partner role and reassure you that the laboring person is all right and behaving normally
- Begin arranging the room, bringing in equipment for the birth, setting up the warmer for the baby (see page 163)

This is an exciting moment, when everyone begins preparing for the infant. At last, even the staff act as if a baby is really coming!

HOW YOU CAN HELP

Your role during transition is all-important. You can truly relieve some of the laboring person's burden if you know what to do:

- Help the laboring person maintain or resume the rhythmic ritual (see page 55). With all these challenges, it helps to know that transition is much more manageable if the laboring person has developed a spontaneous rhythmic ritual earlier in the labor. You can help them return to the familiar.
- If the laboring person is panicky and afraid, use the Take-Charge routine (see page 86). This may be the most important way you can help them resume their ritual.
- Stop worrying about relaxation during contractions. It is unrealistic to expect the laboring person to relax when labor is this intense.
- Stay calm. Keep your touch firm and confident and your voice calm and encouraging. Maintain a confident expression on your face (not worried or pitying).
- Stay close to the laboring person, with your face near theirs.
- Remind them that this difficult phase is short and that the birthing stage is imminent. Help them through one contraction at a time.
- Remind yourself it is normal for the transition phase to be difficult, that the laboring person's mood will improve when the cervix is fully dilated, and that you must not worry. Their behavior is not abnormal and the pain is not more than one should expect at this time.
- If the laboring person wants to avoid pain medications (see "Pain Medications Preference Scale," pages 145–146), do not mention them. Instead, help the laboring person get through this phase without them, as tough as it may be. If, however, they cannot maintain any rhythm and seem panicky, even though you and others are helping all you can, and the nurse or midwife says it will be some time before the baby arrives, this might be a good time to consider pain medication or for you to give a reminder the about the code word (see page 147). If they do not use the code word, continue to help them cope without pain medications.
- If the nurse or caregiver isn't in the room when the laboring person has an urge to push, summon help immediately. The caregiver will observe the laboring person's behavior or check the cervix to determine whether pushing is appropriate.
- If the caregiver says it isn't time to push yet (because the cervix isn't fully dilated), help the laboring person avoid pushing or push with little grunts (see page 41).
- Try not to take it personally if the laboring person criticizes you or tells you to stop doing something you expected to be helpful. Just say, "Sorry," and stop doing it. Don't try to explain why you did it or express frustration. You are just being told that labor is so difficult right now that nothing helps. You are the safest person to lash out at.

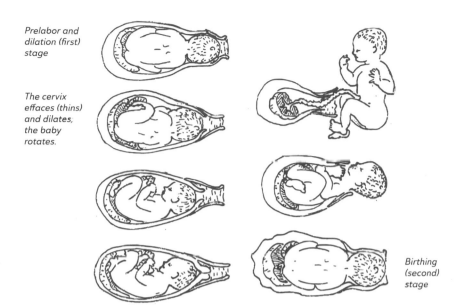

Prelabor and dilation (first) stage

The cervix effaces (thins) and dilates, the baby rotates.

Birthing (second) stage

The baby's head enters the vaginal canal; there may be a "rest" while the uterus tightens around the baby's body; the baby descends and rotates and then is born.

THE BIRTHING, SECOND, STAGE

This stage begins when the cervix is fully dilated and ends with the birth of the baby. During this stage, the baby rotates, descends through the vagina (birth canal), and is born. Medical professionals call this the *second stage.*

During the birthing stage, the birthing person works very hard, bearing down—actively pushing—by holding their breath and straining or breathing out forcefully and vocally with the urge to push that comes several times in every contraction. In this way, they work *together* with the uterus to press the baby down and out.

The birthing stage has three distinct phases: resting, descent, and crowning and birth phases. Each phase is characterized by different physical developments and each requires the laboring person to make an emotional adjustment.

Care of the birthing person and baby during the birthing (second) stage varies among caregivers. Some are guided by patience and assessment of the birthing person's and baby's well-being. These caregivers feel it is best to let the birth unfold spontaneously, without interference, if the birthing person and baby are doing well. Instead of rushing the birthing person to push, these caregivers await the birthing person's spontaneous urge. The caregiver may encourage breathing through the contractions and bearing down when the urge to push compels them to do so. If the resting phase lasts a long time, the caregiver may encourage the birthing person to change positions.

Other caregivers are not as patient. They want to speed the baby's descent as much as possible and so coach the birthing person to push (holding their breath and straining) during contractions while they count to 10. Then, they instruct to quickly take another breath and push for 10 more counts and to repeat this pattern until the contraction ends. These caregivers tend to place a time limit on the second stage (usually 2 hours or fewer for a first-time labor and 1 hour for the second or later births) and use drugs, instruments, and episiotomy to meet this limit.

HOW LONG DOES THE BIRTHING STAGE LAST?
A normal birthing stage may last from 15 minutes (three to five contractions) to 3 hours or more. For most first-time birth-givers, the birthing stage is completed in up to 3 hours; for most people who have given birth before, in less than 1 hour. A longer birthing stage may be due to the position of the baby's head in the pelvis. One possible side effect of an epidural is a greater chance of a malpositioned baby at this time (see page 140). Also, some babies need time for the gradual molding of their head or for tucking the chin and wiggling or rotating into the best-fitting position. Other reasons for a prolonged birthing stage are described on page 129.

The Resting Phase
The resting phase is an apparent pause in the labor. Although not all laboring people experience this phase, you and the person in labor should be ready for it.

The resting phase is a "catch-up break" for the uterus; it comes after the cervix is completely dilated and the baby's head has passed through the cervix into the birth canal. The uterus had been tightly stretched around the baby before the head slipped out. Now, suddenly, only the baby's body remains inside the uterus, and the uterus fits more loosely around the baby. The uterus needs time to tighten around the rest of the baby (see illustration, page 43).

During this phase, the muscle fibers in the uterus shorten, making the uterus smaller, without noticeable contractions and without having an urge to push. After the tumult of transition, the resting phase provides a welcome break. The late Sheila Kitzinger, a famous childbirth educator and prolific author, termed this the "rest-and-be-thankful phase." Birthing persons become alert and clear thinking after the tumult of transition. One person whom Penny worked with looked up at her partner during this phase and asked, "Did you feed the cats?" Only 10 minutes before she had been moaning and tensing during contractions. (Incidentally, he had fed the cats.)

HOW LONG DOES THE RESTING PHASE LAST?
The resting phase usually lasts from 10 to 30 minutes. If it lasts longer than that, the caregiver may ask the person in labor to change position or to try pushing (bearing down), in the hope this will bring on stronger contractions or an urge to push and so speed the labor along. Some caregivers are more patient than others at this time if the baby is doing well, as indicated by the baby's heart rate. Others don't want labor to slow down at this point.

WHAT THE CAREGIVER DOES

During the resting phase:

- The midwife or nurse remains close by, offering encouragement, praise, and positive suggestions.
- The nurse will probably call the doctor to come soon. If the birthing person has had a child before, the doctor will try to arrive soon after pushing begins. If this is a first child, the doctor will probably not rush.
- The midwife or nurse may become more directive at this time, telling the birthing person what positions to try or coaching how or when to push.
- The midwife or nurse listens frequently to the baby's heartbeat and continues assessing the birthing person's welfare.
- The midwife or nurse may do a vaginal exam to assess the progress of the baby's descent.
- The midwife or nurse may apply warm compresses on the perineum to help relax the pelvic floor muscles and improve their sense of how and where to push. The midwife may also pour some oil over the perineum to lubricate the vaginal outlet.

HOW YOU CAN HELP

The birthing stage is an exciting time. Even though you have your own powerful emotional reaction to the birth, if you are the birthing person's major source of support, you must remain calm and continue to encourage and assist. Here are some guidelines:

- Be patient during the resting phase. Don't rush the birthing person through it or make them push too soon.
- If the nurse or caregiver wants the birthing person to push without a contraction or an urge to push, ask whether it can wait until they feel the urge.
- Match the birthing person's mood. As they leave the emotions of transition behind, you do the same.
- If you are confused, ask the midwife, nurse, or doula what is happening.

The Descent Phase

This phase is the longest of the three phases of the birthing stage. During the descent phase, the uterus resumes contracting strongly, and the birthing person usually feels an increasingly strong urge to push. The baby descends through the birth canal to the point where the top of the head is clearly visible at the vaginal outlet. The birthing person alternately pushes and breathes lightly during contractions and rests between contractions.

By *pushing*, we mean that the birthing person takes in a breath and strains (bears down) for 5 to 6 seconds at a time. While bearing down, they either hold their breath or let air out with a moan or bellow. The pushing may be directed, which means they push when told, regardless of whether there is an urge; this technique is used for people who have had epidurals, as they usually feel no urge to push. Or, the pushing can be spontaneous, which means the birthing person bears down with the reflexive urge to push. By this time, a rhythmic ritual is no longer possible or desirable, as the birthing person's behavior is being guided by their reflexive pushing urges, which come three or four times over the peak of each contraction. The urges last about 5 or 6 seconds, with 3 to 5 seconds in between.

Many birthing people tell us that the term *urge to push* does not come close to describing the feeling. One woman cried out during this stage, "It's like a vomit in reverse!" That, crude as it is, is a much better description. The urge to push can be as involuntary and as uncontrollable as vomiting, except that all the force moves downward instead of upward (and the result is a lot more rewarding!).

Sometimes, especially early in the descent phase, the urge to push is a much milder sensation, like a catch in the breath and a grunting sensation. Occasionally, a person who hasn't had an epidural lacks the urge to push. They may simply be having a long resting phase; a change of position and some patience usually result in an urge to push. Or perhaps, the uterus is not contracting with enough intensity to bring on an urge to push; synthetic oxytocin might be used in such a case. If the birthing person is having good contractions and no urge to push, the caregiver instructs when to push.

It can take a few minutes to an hour or two of pushing before the baby's head is visible at the vaginal opening. Before it becomes visible, there is progress in rotation and molding of the baby's head and some descent, but these changes are undetectable from the outside. It can seem as if nothing is happening, but your job is to remain optimistic and supportive, knowing that changes are happening on the inside.

Then, the birthing person's perineum bulges with bearing down. Soon thereafter, the labia part and the tiny vaginal outlet gradually enlarges as the baby moves down. Next, the head becomes visible, though at first it looks more like a wrinkled walnut. The walnut seems to grow bigger with the bearing-down efforts. But rather than moving steadily downward the baby moves down when the birthing person bears down and slips back during the pauses between the bearing-down efforts. If you watch this incredible process, you will likely find yourself totally engrossed. You almost hate to see the baby slip back each time because you're so eager to see them born. You must remember that progress is being made, and this gradual stretching is easier on both baby and birthing person than constant pressure on the baby's head and continuous stretching of the vagina.

The birthing person may change positions during the descent phase. The most common positions are semi-reclining, lying flat on one's back, side lying, on hands and knees, and squatting. Supported squatting, lap squatting, "the dangle," and sitting on the toilet are also useful at times. See "Positions and Movements for Labor and Birth," pages 67–76, for illustrations of each of these positions and descriptions of their benefits.

HOW LONG DOES THE DESCENT PHASE LAST?

The descent phase usually takes up most of the total time of the birthing stage—from a few minutes to as long as 4 hours. The average is about 1½ hours.

WHAT THE CAREGIVER DOES

During the descent phase:

- The midwife or nurse continues as before, encouraging the birthing person's efforts and offering reassurance. This may include coaching the birthing person to breathe lightly during the contraction until the urge to push is stronger and then coaching them to hold their breath and strain.
- The doctor usually arrives during this phase, sometimes to everyone's great relief.
- The doctor, midwife, or nurse performs occasional vaginal exams to confirm the baby's progress through the birth canal. They check the baby's heart rate and the birthing person's vital signs periodically.
- When birth is imminent, they scrub their hands and don surgical gloves, special hospital clothing, and a mask.
- They may place drapes beneath the laboring person, cleanse the vaginal area, and massage the perineum or place warm compresses on it.
- Many caregivers, including most midwives, are in favor of the birthing person using many positions— side lying, hands and knees, semi-reclining, or others (see illustrations of positions for labor and birth, pages 67–76). However, some caregivers prefer that the birthing person be on their back with their legs in stirrups for pushing and/or the birth. If so, the nurse, doctor, or midwife prepares the bed for delivery by removing the foot section and placing the birthing person's legs in supports attached to each side of the bed. They then sit close to the birthing person's perineum. This setup is helpful if medical assistance is needed for the birth (with forceps, a vacuum extractor, and/or an episiotomy), but many doctors prefer it for all births. It is uncomfortable and restrictive for most birthing people. If the birthing person prefers not to be in this position unless necessary, say so in the birth plan.
- The doctor or midwife uses their hands to control the emergence of the baby's head.

HOW YOU CAN HELP

If there are more people around during the descent phase, you may feel less vital to the birthing person than you felt earlier. It is true that they now receive much of the direction and praise from the professionals. This may be a relief as it allows you to become absorbed in your own experience of the birth. You are, however, still the birth partner—the one who has seen the birthing person through this—and they still may rely on you despite all the attention from others.

Suggestions to consider:

- Don't leave at this time if you want to see the baby's birth. Things can change quickly.
- Stay close to the birthing person, where they can see, feel, and hear you. You may support from behind or by their side.
- Don't try to keep a rhythm now because the urge to push takes over and they must respond to that.
- Praise them on how well they are doing—after every contraction.
- Mop their brow and neck with a cold washcloth. Pushing is hard, sweaty work!

- Stay calm. Maintain a steady, reassuring tone of voice and a confident, firm touch. (Don't rub or squeeze too hard in your excitement.)
- Do not tell the birthing person to push harder; you only make them feel inadequate. Instead, offer encouragement like, "That's the way! Come on, Baby."
- Help the birthing person get in and out of positions for pushing, such as squatting or hands and knees, or the less common dangle or lap squatting (see page 75). If they're on their side or semisitting, hold a leg up (someone else will need to hold the other leg; see page 70).
- If progress is slow, be patient; suggest a different position and help the birthing person change positions every 30 minutes, or more often, if needed. Be ready to support them in these positions.
- Using whatever suggestions work, remind them to relax the perineum: "Let go," "Relax your bottom," "Let the baby out." You might remind them to relax the same way as during perineal massage (see page 80).
- Request warm compresses to be placed on the perineum.
- Remind the birthing person that the baby is almost here! Sometimes, believe it or not, they almost forget this is all for the baby.
- Remember that during the first few contractions after the baby's head becomes visible at the vaginal opening, the head may appear wrinkled and spongy. One birth partner thought he was seeing a brain without a skull or scalp! Pressure on the head by the vaginal wall squeezes the skin of the scalp toward the top of the head until the head moves down more. Then, it looks more as you expect—hard and smooth, bluish gray, and bald or hairy.
- If the descent phase seems slow, remember that sometimes more time is needed for the baby's head to mold or to get into the best position in the birthing person's pelvis. If you are discouraged, don't let the birthing person know.

The Crowning and Birth Phase

During the crowning and birth phase the baby is born. This phase begins when the baby's head crowns—that is, when it remains visible at the vaginal opening even between contractions, no longer sneaking back between the bearing-down efforts—and ends when the baby is born.

During the crowning and birth phase, the baby's head stretches the vagina and perineum, which may cause feelings of burning and stinging. Because the vaginal and perineal tissues might tear at this time, protecting the perineum now becomes a major focus of the caregiver's role.

Until now, the baby's head has appeared wrinkled and spongy. Once the head crowns, the skin evens out over the scalp. The head seems to lurch forward a few times, and then it emerges—first the top of the head, then the brow and ears, and then the face. The head rotates to one side; one shoulder appears; and the rest of the baby slides out with a gush of water.

The baby may immediately cry and appear vigorous or may appear bluish and lifeless at first. Under normal circumstances, babies begin breathing within seconds usually with a gurgle and then a lusty cry. Immediately, their color begins to turn, and very soon their skin becomes its normal color.

HOW LONG DOES THE CROWNING AND BIRTH PHASE LAST?

The crowning and birth phase takes only a few contractions.

WHAT THE CAREGIVER DOES

During the crowning and birth phase, the caregiver:

- Supports the perineum and controls the passage of the baby's head as it crowns
- Tells the birthing person to stop pushing as the head emerges, or earlier, when they begin to feel the burning and stretching. The uterus will still contract and there will still be an urge to push. To help avoid a tear, the birthing person should keep from holding their breath and straining as much as possible. To do this, they raise their chin and blow lightly throughout the contraction (see "Avoiding Forceful Pushing," page 64).
- May consider doing an episiotomy (see page 118 for a discussion of this uncommon procedure)
- Holds the baby's head as it emerges; the caregiver may encourage both of you to touch or even hold the baby during the actual birth.
- Dries and places the baby skin to skin on the birthing person's abdomen or in a heated crib nearby, depending on the caregiver's routine, the baby's condition, and your preference

A nurse or doctor checks the baby quickly and gives an Apgar score (see page 106) at 1 minute of age and again at 5 minutes. Five signs are evaluated in order to decide whether the baby needs extra immediate care, close observation, or no extra attention at all. A total score of 7 points or above is very good. If the score is below 7 at 1 minute, the baby may need extra observation and care. By 5 minutes, problems such as sluggish movement, slow pulse, or uneven breathing are usually corrected with stimulation or an oxygen mask.

HOW YOU CAN HELP

During the crowning and birth phase, you can help the birthing person in the following ways:

- Stay close by.
- Help with their position by holding a leg, lifting their shoulders for pushing, or letting them lean on you in a squatting position; see pages 67–76 for illustrations of positions for pushing and ways to support a person while pushing.
- If the midwife or doctor tells the birthing person to stop pushing so as not to injure their body or the baby with too rapid a delivery, the birthing person may find it difficult to comply. Help them avoid pushing by getting them to follow your directions: "Lift your chin, look at me, blow . . . blow . . . that's the way . . . blow . . ." and so forth.

- Participate in this miracle in the way that is most comfortable for the two of you. Stay at the head of the bed and focus on the birthing person's face if that's where you're needed or if you feel squeamish about watching the baby come out. Or, take it all in by watching in the mirror or by moving so you can watch closely. Please don't get so caught up in the birth that you ignore the birthing person!
- Remember, although the baby's initial appearance may be dusky (bluish) and almost lifeless, it will begin to change within seconds as the baby breathes and cries.

THE PLACENTAL, THIRD, STAGE

The placental stage begins when the baby is born and ends after the placenta, or *after-birth*, is born.

This stage is usually anticlimactic when compared to the baby's birth, and many people barely notice the few contractions and the emergence of the placenta. Others feel sharp cramps. The two phases of the placental stage, the separation of the placenta and the expulsion of the placenta, are usually indistinguishable to the birthing person. Medical professionals call this the *third* stage of labor.

HOW LONG DOES THE PLACENTAL STAGE LAST?

The placental stage is the shortest stage of labor. It usually lasts 15 to 30 minutes.

WHAT THE CAREGIVER DOES

During the placental stage, the caregiver:

- Attends to the umbilical cord, clamping it and either cutting it or inviting the partner to cut it. It is usually best for the baby to wait a few minutes before clamping and cutting the cord (see page 161). The caregiver withdraws some blood from the cord, to analyze for the baby's blood type or, if the parents wish, to donate it or to store it privately in a blood bank. (Umbilical cord blood is a rich source of stem cells that can be used for children or adults with certain cancers or blood disorders, as an alternative to a bone marrow transplant. Consult your caregiver to learn more about this procedure and the options in your area. Also check page 190, Recommended Resources.)
- Dries and checks the baby
- Checks the birthing parent's birth canal to see whether stitches are needed
- Attends to the placenta. When the placenta has separated from the uterine wall (the caregiver can tell by feeling the uterus and putting gentle traction on the cord), they may ask the birthing person to gently push to deliver the placenta.
- Carefully inspects the placenta to make sure all of it has been delivered. If fragments remain in the uterus, the caregiver must remove them by hand (see page 133).
- Palpates the abdomen to feel whether the uterus is firm. If it is "boggy," the nurse or midwife vigorously massages the uterus through the abdominal wall. This is uncomfortable for the birthing person, but is very effective in contracting the uterus and protecting against excessive blood loss. The nurse can teach the birthing person to do this on their own abdomen (see page 159).

HOW YOU CAN HELP

During the placental stage, you can do the following:

- Cut the cord, if you want to; the caregiver will likely invite you to do this. The symbolism of separating the pregnant person and the baby appeals to many new parents and their partners. You may be surprised at how firm and slippery the cord is. When you cut it, don't snip gently; make a decisive effort.
- Enjoy the baby and help the new parent do the same—this is your main role now. Make sure your partner is comfortable, can see the baby, and is warm enough.
- Make sure the baby stays warm. The warmest—and happiest—place for the baby is skin to skin against the birthing parent, with the two of them covered by a warm blanket. Unfortunately, many hospitals customarily keep a baby in a warming unit while the nurse does all the newborn procedures (see page 160). Then, the baby is wrapped and given a hat. If the baby is presented to the new parent all wrapped up, ask whether the baby can be placed naked against their skin with a warm blanket over both. Babies stay perfectly warm when held and covered in this way. Do not leave the baby uncovered or remove the hat unless the room is very warm. If a newborn becomes chilled, it may take a long time (often in the nursery, away from the parents) to return to normal temperature.
- Go along if the baby must go to the nursery (either because of a health problem or because it is hospital policy), unless the birthing parent needs you to stay behind. Soothe the baby by talking and singing their song.
- Jump at the chance, when it's your turn, to hold the baby close. If your partner and baby are both healthy, it's a good idea for them to be together, skin to skin at first, and for you and the baby to get together later in the fourth stage (see following). Talk or sing to the baby and begin getting acquainted. The baby already knows and loves your voice.
- Congratulate yourselves on a job well done and start making those phone calls, as the after-birth care (see chapter 9) of your partner and baby begins.

The Recovery and Bonding, Fourth, Stage

For the birthing person, the fourth stage refers to the first few hours after birth, when the birthing person's condition stabilizes.

If the birth has been without medications or interventions, the birthing person's own oxytocin, which began to surge during the baby's journey down the birth canal, is now at high levels; endorphins are also flowing, and these combine to give the birthing person high spirits and feelings of love and gratefulness. These hormones also help override the fatigue, pain, and discouragement that may have been felt earlier. Epidural analgesia reduces oxytocin and endorphin production, which may moderate the positive feelings.

The baby, during these first hours of life, undergoes an enormous physiological shift from dependency on the pregnant person and placenta for survival and growth to dependence on themselves for such basic survival functions as breathing, taking in food, regulating body temperature, and adapting to the new surroundings. Before birth, the lungs were not important to the baby, so most of the baby's blood bypassed the lungs.

Immediately after birth, however, the structure of the baby's heart changes so all the baby's blood is rerouted through the lungs to pick up oxygen and carry it wherever needed. Within minutes, the birthing parent no longer provides oxygen to the baby, who is now breathing and can get their own oxygen. You will witness these profound changes in the baby if you are present at the birth!

HOW LONG DOES THE RECOVERY AND BONDING STAGE LAST?
This stage usually lasts 2 to 4 hours.

WHAT THE CAREGIVER DOES
The caregiver checks the birthing parent's vital signs (pulse, blood pressure, temperature, respiration rate) and the firmness of the uterus to be sure it remains contracted (which minimizes blood loss). If the uterus is "boggy" or soft, the caregiver massages it to make it contract. This can be quite uncomfortable but is very important to prevent excessive blood loss. Ask the caregiver to show the birthing parent how to do it. They may be able to get a good result without massaging as hard.

The caregiver also checks the perineum to see if the stretching during birth caused damage that requires stitches. If yes, they go ahead with the repair (using local anesthesia, if your partner did not get an epidural or other anesthetic earlier in labor). The caregiver also helps get feeding established, placing the baby skin to skin on the birthing parent's chest. The caregiver also checks the baby's Apgar score, which assesses five vital indicators of the baby's condition to determine whether the baby needs extra medical attention (see page 106 for details on the Apgar score).

HOW YOU CAN HELP
Keeping birthing parent and baby together skin to skin in the first hours after birth, as long as both are healthy, helps get the family off to a good start. Not only is the birthing person providing everything the baby needs—warmth, colostrum, familiar heartbeat and voice, touch stimulation, smell, and more—but the baby reciprocates by stimulating shrinking of the uterus, successful breastfeeding, and bonding.

The baby's actions on the birthing parent's abdomen and nuzzling and suckling at the breast releases oxytocin that stimulates the uterus to contract. These actions also stimulate the birthing parent's pituitary gland to secrete prolactin, the key to both the production of breast milk and to altruistic behavior (i.e., putting the baby's needs ahead of their own), which is essential for the baby's survival. When unrushed and undisturbed, both of you can become acquainted with your child and discover all your baby's little mannerisms and sounds at your own pace.

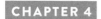

CHAPTER 4

Comfort Measures for Labor

The pain of labor has many physical causes. In the first stage, pain is caused by:

- Contractions of the uterus—the strongest muscle in the human body—which reach maximum intensity during this stage. (Try doing several chin-ups for 1 minute at a time. The muscle pain in your arms is similar to the kind of pain caused by uterine contractions, but less intense.)
- Stretching of the cervix as it opens. (Try sitting on the floor with your legs out straight and bending forward as far as possible with your hands grasping your lower legs. This will give you a sense of the nature of the pain caused by the cervix stretching.)
- Stretching of pelvic ligaments from the pressure of the baby's head within the pelvis. This causes mild to severe back pain. One-fourth to one-third of laboring women have back pain during labor.

In the birthing stage, pain is caused by uterine contractions, pressure in the pelvis, and also by stretching of the pelvic floor muscles, the vaginal canal, and the skin of the vaginal outlet.

Labor pain also can be increased by fear, worry, shame, or exhaustion. These can affect the laboring person as much as physical causes and can turn pain into suffering.

PAIN VERSUS SUFFERING

Although the terms *pain* and *suffering* are often used interchangeably, there is a big difference between the two. Labor, even when long and painful, does not inevitably cause suffering. Pain is an unpleasant physical sensation that may or may not be associated with suffering. For example, the pain people feel when working out at the gym or jogging uphill is not suffering. Consider the motto, "No pain, no gain." Suffering is a distressing psychological state that may include feelings of helplessness, anguish, remorse, fear, panic, or loss of control and may or may not be associated with pain. For example, being jilted by a lover or emotionally abused (ignored, insulted, or humiliated) or witnessing another person being hurt or injured may cause one to suffer, even though one may feel no physical sensation of pain.

Many people tell us that what worries them most about labor pain is they will be overwhelmed, helpless, and out of control. They worry the pain will take them beyond their limits and make them behave in a shameful way. This is a fear of suffering. If they carry this fear into labor, the fear will augment the pain, and they will likely suffer in the ways they fear. These pregnant people do not have confidence that labor pain can be manageable and that it does not inevitably lead to suffering.

When pregnant people recognize that labor pain is really a side effect of a normal process, not a sign of damage or injury, fear cannot increase the pain. Most of us have had pain that we did not understand, and it frightened us. For example, when I (Penny) turned my ankle with an awful crunching sound, I was terrified I had broken it. In great pain, I was rushed to the emergency room where I was told there was no break, only a bad strain that should clear up if I wore a stabilizing boot for a couple of weeks. I immediately felt better and was able to walk (or limp) out of the hospital I had entered in a wheelchair. Once knowledge replaced fear, my pain diminished.

Some laboring people will cross from pain to suffering if they become exhausted or if something interferes with their confidence or way of coping, such as frequent disturbances, rigid hospital routines, thoughtless or demoralizing remarks, lack of emotional support, or clinical complications. If a laboring person understands why contractions hurt and are continuously nurtured and encouraged by humane, caring, confident people in a peaceful and safe environment; if they are free to move about to find greater comfort; and if they know effective ways to respond to contractions, fear gives way to mastery, confidence, and a sense of well-being. Even though the contractions become very intense, the pregnant person does not suffer—they cope.

How to Decrease Pain and Prevent Suffering in Labor

There are many ways you and the laboring person can reduce labor pain. Through childbirth education (classes, this book, video, media, and internet resources), you can learn about the birth process, self-help comfort measures, the wide range of other measures to relieve labor pain, and other options regarding the laboring person's care in labor. Laboring persons can use relaxation techniques, rhythmic breathing or moaning, attention focusing, movements, and positions. You can help by never leaving them alone in labor, attending to their emotional needs, comforting with massage, hand holding, and hot or cold packs, by suggesting a shower or bath, and by assisting them in the use of other self-help comfort measures, which we discuss here.

This chapter tells you more specifically what you can do to ease the laboring person's pain. These numerous techniques do not take away all pain, but, when combined with caring and skilled labor support, they enable many people in labor to cope successfully with the pain. Some people in labor use these techniques in combination with pain-relieving medications; others rely on the techniques alone.

Make sure, before labor begins, that you know and respect the pregnant person's preferences regarding the use of pain medications. Use the "Pain Medications Preference Scale," pages 145–146, to help describe their feelings and whether your feelings are different. Then, you will know how to react if and when they approach their pain tolerance limits. You will either ask for pain medication (see chapter 8) or redouble your efforts in encouraging, guiding, and helping the laboring person continue to handle the pain. For the latter, many of the comfort measures described here are highly effective.

The techniques described in this chapter work in different ways, by:

- Eliminating or reducing factors causing the pain
- Increasing other pleasant or neutral sensations to dampen the awareness of pain
- Involving the laboring person in activities that focus attention on something other than the pain
- Showing the laboring person they are cared for, respected, and heard

Using a variety of techniques seems more helpful than doing the same thing for the entire labor.

Learn the following techniques before labor so you can suggest them when appropriate and help the laboring person use them. Along with the lists in chapter 1, the information in this chapter will also help you choose comfort items to take to the hospital (or have ready in your home) to use during labor.

As you learn these techniques and positions, keep in mind there are other ways to help a person through labor. Sometimes, the best thing to do is simply to be there, quietly standing by, while labor unfolds and the laboring person searches within for the best way to respond. If they seem withdrawn and incommunicative, do not be concerned. You don't need to engage them in discussion. Let them discover what they need from you. Take your lead from them in the moment rather than trying to plan it all in advance.

THE THREE RS: RELAXATION, RHYTHM, AND RITUAL

Coping well with the pain and indeterminate length of labor involves the use of the Three Rs: relaxation, rhythm, and ritual. The concept of the Three Rs arose from my (Penny's) observations as a doula for hundreds of laboring women. I learned some people cope well with pain and stress in labor; others are overwhelmed. I noticed these three responses to contractions are shared by most people who cope well:

- The person can relax during or between contractions or both. Relaxation often involves remaining still, with limp limbs (passive relaxation) while breathing slowly and fully. It really helps reduce discomfort if the laboring person releases tension, remains still, and goes limp throughout the body. Alternatively, it is also soothing and relaxing to sway, rock, moan, chant, or sing rhythmically. This is called "active relaxation" and can be very helpful, especially with the intense contractions of later labor or if passive relaxation is no longer doable. Between contractions, the laboring person rests or resumes normal activity until the next contraction.
- The use of rhythm to cope
- The discovery and use of rituals—personally meaningful rhythmic activities repeated with every contraction

Using Rituals During Labor

In prelabor and very early labor, a laboring person coping well uses distracting activities until the contractions become intense enough they can no longer continue walking or talking through them. When they must stop everything for 30 seconds or so at each contraction's peak, the laboring person stops trying to use distraction and begins using a ritual.

During early labor, the ritual is usually one rehearsed in advance, perhaps in childbirth class. If they haven't learned a ritual in advance, the nurse or doula may teach one in the moment. This "planned" ritual usually involves sighing (breathing slowly, audibly, and rhythmically), releasing muscle tension with each exhale, and focusing attention in some positive way (for example, letting go of tension in one muscle group at a time: brow, shoulders, arms, buttocks, legs or counting breaths through the contractions).

As labor intensifies, the laboring person may adopt another planned ritual. They may change to a lighter, quicker, rhythm of breathing (4 to 6 shallow breaths every 10 seconds), move rhythmically (sway, rock, slow dance with you, their partner, [see page 170], or tap or stroke themselves, you, a pillow, or other object), and focus their attention by staring into your face, counting their breaths, using imagery, or chanting, singing, moaning, or self-talking, audibly or not.

By this time in labor (around 5 centimeters in dilation), however, many laboring people stop thinking and behave more instinctually as they give up trying to control the labor. Their planned ritual gives way as they discover their own spontaneous rituals. These become very powerful aids in getting through each contraction. Once laboring people discover these rituals, they repeat them for many contractions. Then, as labor changes, they may change rituals spontaneously once again.

What do labor rituals have in common? As already described, they always seem to involve rhythm in some way. In fact, rhythm is the most essential element in the Three Rs. Sometimes, the rhythm is supplied by someone or something else, in the form of murmuring, rhythmic stroking or pressure, pouring water over the contracting belly, or moaning or swaying together.

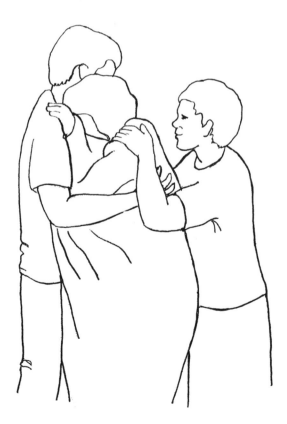

How to Help with Labor Rituals

As birth partner, you can help a laboring person develop or continue their ritual. First, observe their behavior during contractions. Are they still, with relaxed muscles? Or, are they moving or vocalizing in a rhythm? If doing any of these, they are coping well, even if the ritual involves moaning loudly or swaying vigorously. If they have lost the rhythm, your job (or the doula's) is to help them find or regain a rhythm (see "The Take-Charge Routine," page 86, and "How You Can Help," page 39). Do not interrupt the ritual during a contraction by asking a question or suggesting some other approach.

Your assistance will probably be more active with the use of an external ritual than an internal ritual. For example, with an external ritual you might:

- Maintain eye contact
- Help keep a rhythm by moving your head or hands, stroking, or murmuring soothing words in the rhythm of their breathing or moaning
- Press firmly on their upper arms, hands, thighs, or feet to anchor them
- Press on their hips or low back
- Hold them close, walk, sway, or slow dance together
  If they use an internal ritual, you might:
- Remain close by, holding their hand quietly and calmly
- Refrain from, and ask others to refrain from, disturbing them during contractions
- If you have prepared for a very active support role, you may feel useless if the laboring person uses an internal ritual. You may want to do more, to have them look at you or allow you to stroke or talk to them. You must realize, however, they need you, but more as a calm, caring presence than an active helper. If they are coping (relaxing during contractions and remaining still, with eyes closed), engaging with eye contact or following your rhythm will be disruptive.

Even if the laboring person does not seem to need much help from you at the moment, continue to observe and be in their rhythm during contractions (see Resources, "Aids for Relaxation, page 190). If they begin to wince or tense or vocalize or lose rhythm, get their attention and help them regain the rhythm.

If there are continual interruptions—examinations by a nurse or caregiver, checking their pulse, taking their temperature or blood pressure, drawing blood, general monitoring—the laboring person may become too unsettled to be able to keep a rhythm or regain their ritual. In this case, you might tell the nurse, "If they could get through a few contractions without interruption, I think they could feel more in control. Is this possible?" If the procedures cannot be postponed, you may need to play a more active "coaching" role. Use the Take-Charge routine (see page 86) and tell the laboring person, "All that matters during this contraction is that you keep your rhythm. Let me help you through this." Help them with their rhythm until they have some quiet, undisturbed time to resume or develop another ritual.

Once the cervix dilates completely and the laboring person is in the birthing stage, they will become more alert and focused. They are less likely to use the same ritual now, and their rhythm will give way to the powerful urge to push. The contractions will now dictate whether, when, and how they push, and they will approach birth in a crescendo of emotion, excitement, and sensation. Instead of helping maintain a ritual during the birthing stage, help them maintain a good position for birth and encourage them to relax the perineum during pushes (see "The Birthing Stage," page 43).

SELF-HELP COMFORT MEASURES

Self-help comfort measures are skills the pregnant person masters before labor to help manage pain and enhance labor progress. Many are taught in childbirth classes, on audio or video media, online streaming sites such as YouTube, or in books. Plan to learn and use these. They can make the difference between feeling overwhelmed by the pain and coping in a positive way. This section covers many self-help comfort measures. Practice them together and adapt them to work best for the pregnant person.

Relaxation

Relaxation, rhythmic breathing, and attention focusing have long been the cornerstones of childbirth preparation. Relaxation is the goal of most comfort measures. If a laboring person lets their body go limp during contractions (passive relaxation) or if they sway, rock, moan, or murmur rhythmically (active relaxation), they will feel less pain or be less overwhelmed. The laboring person's attempt to relax, even if not completely successful, is helpful in itself because it serves as a positive focus away from the pain.

In active labor, passive relaxation during contractions may be more difficult than in early labor; the laboring person may need to keep moving in rhythm. At this phase, the goal is to relax passively between contractions and carry on an active ritual (see page 55) during them.

During the last weeks of pregnancy, help the pregnant person learn to recognize and release tension in all parts of their body. By practicing with them, you learn what tone of voice, which words, and what sort of touch helps them relax. Try the following:

- While the pregnant person lies still, as they breathe slowly and deeply, state which body parts to focus on and relax. Start at the toes and gradually go through the parts of the body up to the head.
- Help the pregnant person identify any "tension spots" and release the tension at will. A tension spot is a part of the body where tension seems to settle when they are stressed. This same spot (or spots) is likely to be the seat of tension during labor. Tension spots might be the shoulders, neck, brow, jaw, low back, or buttocks. Help them let go of tension when you touch the spot with your whole hand or when you say, for example, "Relax your right shoulder," or "Let go right here." If the pregnant person has difficulty relaxing, they can learn to let a particular part of their body go limp by first tensing it (for example, tightening the arm or leg as much as possible) and then relaxing it. Repeating this exercise trains both of you to recognize when their body is tense and trains the pregnant person to relax.

Good childbirth preparation classes emphasize passive and active relaxation techniques. DVDs and YouTube videos are also available to help people master the skill of relaxation for childbirth. See Recommended Resources (page 190) for a description of some helpful aids for relaxation.

During labor, you can help the laboring person relax in the following ways:

- When they feel a contraction start, remind them to begin their ritual immediately (if they don't do it spontaneously), using rhythmic exhales to release tension. Remind them that each exhale is a relaxing breath.
- If you notice tension in any part of their body as the contraction intensifies, use soothing words or touch (or both) to help them let go of tension in those places. Don't just say, "Relax." Be more specific. Instead say, "Let go right here," as you touch a hands, brow, shoulder, and so forth. Your touch should be comforting, not tense or tentative. When they releasing tension, say, "Good," or "Just like that."
- Use the comfort measures in this chapter and verbal reminders to help the laboring person relax during and between contractions. Trial and error will tell you what works best. Once you find something that works, stick with it.
- If labor becomes so intense that the laboring person is unable to relax during contractions despite your efforts, help them relax and rest between contractions while keeping a rhythm during them. Use soothing words, touch, and other comfort measures.

Attention Focusing

This technique diverts the laboring person's mind from the pain by having them concentrate on something else. During contractions, attention can be refocused in several ways:

- The laboring woma can look at you or a meaningful picture, figurine, flowers, or another object. One person hung a baby's outfit on the wall and focused on it and the fact that they soon would fill the suit with a baby. Another person made an inspiring collage to hang on the birthing room wall, it included beautiful scenery and images of powerful people doing impressive physical and artistic feats. Another posted pictures of her older child's artwork. Still another hung pictures of her many pets—her horse, three dogs, and a cat. All these laboring women used objects to ground or inspire them. Focusing on an object can become an all-important part of a laboring person's ritual.
- The laboring person can listen to your voice, to music, or another soothing sound. Many people like to hear rhythmic murmuring with each contraction.
- They can focus on feeling your touch, your massage, or your caress. Match their rhythm with your stroking.
- They can concentrate on a mantra or mental ritual such as counting breaths or repeating words throughout each contraction. For example, they might chant, "Ooopen . . . , ooopen . . . , ooopen . . ." or say, "I think I can . . . , I think I can . . . , I thought I could . . . , I thought I could. . . ." (from The Little Engine That Could); or repeat, "Be still like the

mountain and flow like the river." One laboring person even loudly repeated the word epidural over and over while swaying through the contractions. The doula asked if they needed an epidural was needed. The person replied, "No, if I can say it, I don't need it!" Usually, these rituals are unplanned and emerge spontaneously. You might join them if they are counting, chanting, or moaning aloud. Certainly, whatever you do, do not interrupt their rhythm. Help them maintain it.

Visualization

The laboring person can visualize something positive, pleasant, or relaxing, using the contractions, focus, or breathing as a cue. For example, they might visualize their exhalations or your soothing touch or massage as drawing the tension and pain away. They might imagine being in a special, safe, comfortable place, where the contractions are cues to relax more deeply into the comfort of the place. They might visualize each contraction in various ways: as a wave and floating over the crest or as a mountain, climbing up and down as the contractions come and go. They might use the onset of the contraction as a cue to imagine soaring like a seagull above the waves of contractions below. Several people from our childbirth classes have told us that during labor they visualized the opening of the cervix of the knitted argyle uterus that we use during classes to demonstrate contractions and dilation.

Some visualizations are planned; others emerge spontaneously in labor. Spontaneous visualizations are usually very creative and personally helpful.

Sometimes, couples plan visualizations together during pregnancy, so the partner can guide the laboring person through them during labor. We recommend recalling some positive or empowering experiences you have shared or that they have gone through. Following are guidelines for two personal visualizations: one for early labor and one for active labor.

To plan a visualization for **early labor**:

1. Think of an activity in which the two of you were relaxed and content (for example, a trip or lovely walk you took together, or a delicious meal, or a warm conversation).
2. Recall as many details of that experience as you can.
3. Weave the details into a brief description with a beginning, a middle, and an end. During contractions, you will narrate the visualization, varying the details with each contraction.

For example, one couple had taken a canoe trip early on a cold misty morning. The river was still; the mist was rising; birds were soaring overhead; a ramshackle barn was visible in the distance; a fallen tree partly blocked the river; and so on. In labor, the person was in a large tub and a friend was pouring water over their back in rhythm with their breathing. With each contraction, the partner said, "Now, let's get in the canoe and glide over the contraction. Birds fly overhead. See the barn with the caved-in roof. There is no one else in sight. It's all so still and beautiful. Now, take your rest." The partner varied the details but repeated them often. Later the birthing person said, "My partner took me back there. My breathing became the strokes of my paddle. The sound of the water being poured over my back became the drips off the paddle when I took it out of the water."

For **active labor**:

1. Ask the pregnant person to describe a time they were challenged—physically, mentally, or artistically—and met that challenge.
2. Weave the event into a brief description that can be narrated during contractions as a reminder of their ability to meet challenges.
3. Plan to vary or intensify the description as labor becomes more intense.

For example, one person recalled regularly riding a bicycle on a trail that had one very steep, long uphill stretch. For a long time, they were unable to make it to the top without walking the bike partway. With persistence, though, they could eventually pedal to the top before coasting down the other side. In active labor, they pictured each contraction as that hill and recalled the persistence it took, with shortness of breath and aching muscles, to get to the top. Their mantra became, "Keep it up. Keep it up." The partner encouraged the laboring person by repeating the mantra and then, "Almost there—a little more—that's right. Now you're over the top. Coast your way down." The laboring person said later that each hill became higher and tougher to climb as the contractions intensified, but the memory of successfully pedaling up the hill helped with every contraction.

Rhythmic Breathing and Moaning

Every method of childbirth preparation has used rhythmic breathing as its mainstay. It is the most widely used comfort technique for childbirth. In a large U.S. survey, 49 percent of laboring people who responded used breathing techniques. A large Canadian survey found that 74 percent used breathing. In fact, success in every demanding physical activity, or sport, as well as meditation and stress-reduction techniques, requires breath awareness and rhythm. Rhythmic breathing or moaning (which is actually vocal breathing), along with relaxation, have tremendous value and offer unique pain relieving capabilities:

- Breathing or moaning in steady rhythm helps one relax, especially when having learned to release tension with each exhalation.
- Rhythmic breathing or moaning is calming, especially when a person feels anxious or overwhelmed.
- Rhythmic breathing or moaning gives the person some measure of control over their responses to the contractions, even though the uterus, with its involuntary and all-encompassing contractions, is completely outside one's conscious control.
- When institutional policy or the laboring person's own condition does not permit comfort measures such as a bath or shower, massage or movement, rhythmic breathing or moaning is always available. (Many comfort measures are impossible, for example, when the person cannot get out of bed, if electronic fetal monitor belts or an intravenous line are in the way, or they have received pain medications; see "When the Birthing Person Must Labor in Bed," page 99, for specific suggestions for such circumstances.)

The laboring person will be able to use breathing rhythms most effectively and with the least effort during labor if the techniques are mastered beforehand.

There are two basic breathing rhythms to use during the dilation (first) stage: *slow breathing and light breathing*. We suggest that you and the pregnant person learn each, adapt their speed and rhythm so you feel comfortable with them, and use them during labor. The laboring person's preferences and the nature of the contractions should guide the two of you in deciding how and when to use these rhythms.

SLOW BREATHING OR MOANING

We suggest beginning with slow rather than light quick breaths because this is the easier of the two rhythms. Start this when distracting activities no longer keep the laboring person comfortable; that is, when contractions become so intense that the laboring person stops in their tracks and is unable to continue walking, talking, or whatever they are doing, through each contraction. From this point, they should use slow breathing for as long as they can relax well with it, perhaps moaning or sighing audibly with each exhale.

For slow breathing to be most relaxing and calming, the key is for the laboring person to breathe easily and fully and not work to keep it slow: "Easy in, easy out." If they are working too hard, their breathing will sound tense and strained and their bodies will show tension.

This is how to use slow breathing during labor:

1. When the contraction begins, the laboring person focuses their attention as described on page 59.
2. They take a big, relaxing sigh, releasing tension throughout the body and, if desired, make a low moaning sound as they breathe out.
3. They breathe in slowly—preferably (though not necessarily) breathing in through the nose and breathing out through the mouth—with each exhale a long sigh or moan. At the end of each exhale, they pause and wait a moment, rather than rushing to inhale. The rate should be somewhere between 5 and 12 breaths per minute. With each exhale, they relax, releasing tension all over or from a different part of the body (such as the brow, jaw, shoulders, or right or left arm). Some people find it relaxing on each exhale to make "horse lips" sounds, which horses sometimes make by letting their loose lips vibrate as they breathe out through their mouths, also called a "nicker."
4. When the contraction ends, normal activity resumes and you do not think about the breathing.

The laboring person should use slow breathing for as long as it helps. Some people use only slow breathing throughout the entire labor. For most, however, the contractions become too intense and close together to maintain the slow breathing. In that case, switch to light breathing. If the laboring person switches to light breathing early in labor, they might be able to return to slow breathing later.

LIGHT BREATHING

Mastering the light breathing rhythm takes some practice, just as it takes time to learn to breathe rhythmically while swimming the crawl stroke. And, just as rhythmic breathing when swimming enables one to swim better, the light breathing rhythm enables the laboring person to manage pain better. (Light breathing is much easier to master than breathing while swimming.) Once mastered, light breathing is as easy to do as slow breathing. This is how to use light breathing during labor:

1. When the contraction begins, the laboring person focuses their attention.
2. They begin breathing in short, light breaths through their mouth, with a silent inhale, an audible exhale, and a brief pause after each exhale. The rate is about 1 breath every 1 or 2 seconds or 30 to 60 breaths per minute. With each exhale, they breathe out tension.
3. The breathing continues at this rate until the contraction begins to subside. Then, they either slow their breathing rate, if desired, or continue at the same light breathing rate until the contraction is over.
4. When the contraction ends, they can rest or resume whatever they were doing before it started. With the next contraction, they repeat the light breathing.

Encourage the pregnant person to practice this rhythm enough to master it before labor starts. It requires only a few practice sessions. At first, light breathing may be uncomfortable (it may cause dry mouth, lightheadedness, or a feeling of not being able to get enough air). By adapting it and working with it, however, the person can become relaxed and comfortable doing it. Light breathing may become their best friend in labor (besides you).

Practice light breathing until the pregnant person is able to breathe at the rate of 30 to 60 breaths per minute for a full 1 to 2 minutes without stopping or feeling lightheaded (from hyperventilating). If they feel lightheaded, slow the pace slightly, pause a bit longer at the end of each breath, or breathe more shallowly (so as not to move as much air in and out). The lightheadedness is annoying and uncomfortable, and it will not occur once the technique is mastered. If the pregnant person masters light breathing before labor begins it is very unlikely they will hyperventilate during labor.

As the pregnant person practices rhythmic breathing, see that they relax all over, especially in the shoulders and trunk. If tense, it is more likely they'll hyperventilate. Remind them to relax. It is helpful if you "entrain" yourself to them by being "in their rhythm." If you sway, bob your head, count their breaths, or move your hand up and down in the rhythm of their breathing, it seems to help them continue in that steady rhythm. Keep your hand and wrist relaxed and floppy while conducting, remembering to stop briefly at the end of each exhale. Your own relaxation is contagious and will help them relax.

Once light breathing without hyperventilating is mastered, the laboring person will be able to adapt these breathing rhythms during labor in whatever way is most comfortable. They may want to combine slow and light breathing; for example, they might begin and end the contraction with slow breathing and use light breathing over the peak.

Do remember, however, that rhythmic breathing is most beneficial if the laboring person can use it easily—without thinking much about it and without tensing. Rhythmic breathing should be relaxing; it becomes an attention-focusing aid in itself once the pregnant person has mastered it.

Pushing (Bearing-Down) Techniques

There are four techniques for handling the urge to push:

- One is used to help the laboring person avoid forceful pushing (or bearing down) when this would be nonproductive or harmful.
- The others are used during the birthing stage, when the birthing person should be pushing; they are spontaneous bearing down, self- directed pushing, and directed pushing.

AVOIDING FORCEFUL PUSHING

There are three occasions during labor when the birthing person should *not* push (holding their breath and straining) even though they feel like doing so. These are:

1. Before the cervix has completely dilated, as determined by a vaginal exam.
   A premature urge to push sometimes happens as early as 6 centimeters, if the baby's head is positioned so that it puts pressure on the vaginal wall.
2. During transition (between 8 and 10 centimeters dilation), if there is still a firm lip, or rim, of cervix remaining (see page 41). The caregiver detects this with a vaginal exam.
3. During the birthing stage, as the baby's head crowns and emerges.

Forceful pushing during dilation or transition might increase the pressure of the baby against the cervix, cause the cervix to swell, and, thus, slow the progress of labor. With a strong urge to push long before the cervix dilates, changing to the open knee–chest position or side- lying position may help (see page 72). During transition, until the lip disappears, the laboring person should push only enough to satisfy the urge (see "Transition," page 41).

If the laboring person is told not to push because of a lip, "grunt pushing" can help keep them from straining too hard. Grunt pushes are quick but gentle breath holds followed by forceful releases of air, which make a grunting sound. You might talk them through each contraction, helping them breathe or do grunt pushes.

During the crowning and birth stage, pushing hard might cause stretching that is too rapid and injures the vagina or a delivery that is too rapid. The laboring person can avoid holding their breath at this time by raising their chin and blowing or panting lightly whenever they feel the urge to push. This is sometimes easier said than done because the urge can be very strong. You can help by keeping eye contact and breathing with them, talking them through it, or nodding your head in the rhythm of their panting.

Don't expect too much from these techniques; they do not take away or diminish the birthing person's urge to push. All they do is minimize additional pushing in excess of what their body is already doing.

SPONTANEOUS BEARING DOWN

Once the birthing person feels like pushing and the cervix is fully dilated, the caregiver will give the go-ahead. Usually, the birthing person should push spontaneously. Spontaneous bearing down works like this:

1. The contraction begins. The birthing person focuses their attention as described on page 59.
2. They use whichever breathing rhythm—slow or light—seems best, until the urge to push is so strong they cannot resist bearing down.
3. The urge to push comes in waves or surges—three to six in each contraction. These surges of the uterus sweep the birthing person along into an involuntary bearing-down effort (holding the breath or grunting, moaning, or straining) that lasts 5 to 7 seconds. Do not worry that they lose rhythm while pushing. In the birthing stage, the urge to push is the guide: rhythm is not important while pushing.
4. Once each surge subsides, they breathe lightly and rhythmically until the next surge. This pattern continues until the contraction is over.
5. When the contraction ends, they rest until the next one.

SELF-DIRECTED PUSHING

This is reserved for times when the birthing person's spontaneous bearing down is ineffective. Their eyes may be clenched shut and they may be wincing, arching their back, tipping their chin up, as if fighting against the contraction. (We sometimes call this diffuse pushing, as the pushing efforts are not directed to move the baby down the birth canal.)

If progress is being made while pushing this way, do not worry. If the baby is not coming down, however, consult the caregiver and try this:

1. Between contractions, tell the laboring person to keep their eyes open and look toward where the baby will come out during the next contraction. This helps focus the pushing efforts downward.
2. You may need to remind them to open their eyes if this seems to improve progress.
3. If there are visible signs of progress, you might hold a mirror so the birthing person can see the baby coming. (Do not be surprised if they do not want to look. This should be their choice.)
4. The laboring person should bear down spontaneously, while looking toward where the baby will emerge.
5. If still bearing down ineffectively, suggest a change of position. Any change of position may help focus and push more effectively.
6. If these measures do not succeed, try directed pushing.

DIRECTED PUSHING

Until the late 1980s, directed pushing was the only bearing-down technique used in virtually every hospital. With this technique, the birthing person would be coached to hold their breath and strain as hard as they could for a count of 10 and then grab a breath and repeat this throughout every contraction. Research has shown that using forceful prolonged breath holding and straining may exhaust the birthing person, cause distress in the baby (because the breath holding decreases oxygen for the baby), and cause extreme stretching of the pelvic floor muscles and ligaments supporting the bladder and uterus, which can lead to later bladder and bowel problems.

Today, directed pushing is used under the following circumstances:

- When the baby's descent is too slow with spontaneous bearing down and the caregiver is considering assisting the delivery with instruments—forceps or a vacuum extractor (see pages 120–121)—or episiotomy (see page 118). The birthing person should try directed pushing before the instruments are used.
- When the birthing person has been given an epidural and cannot fully feel the urge to push and so cannot use the spontaneous bearing-down pattern. In this case, however, some side effects may be eliminated if they can use the modified form of directed pushing described below.
- When directed pushing remains the routine in the institution. Ask the birthing person's caregiver in advance whether the staff advocate spontaneous bearing down or directed pushing.

MODIFIED DIRECTED PUSHING

Except when needed to avoid the use of instruments, the directed-pushing technique can be modified to resemble spontaneous bearing down to reduce undesirable effects:

1. The contraction begins. The birthing person focuses. You, the nurse, or doula says what to do: "Breathe in and out, two to four times, letting the contraction build. Now, hold your next breath and strain—1, 2, 3, 4, 5, 6. Now, breathe for the baby. Take several quick breaths in and out and repeat the breath holding and straining."
2. The birthing person continues in this way until the contraction subsides.
3. The contraction ends. They rest until the next one.

Movement and Position Changes

When free to move and change positions, the birthing person:

- Is more comfortable and labor may even speed up
- Can find positions or movements that feel right
- May stand, walk, sit, recline, squat, kneel, lie on one side, get on hands and knees, or lean on you, the wall, a birth ball, the bed, or the nightstand (see illustrations, page 169)
- May walk, rock, or sway rhythmically

Encourage the birthing person to try a change in position or movement if they are restless, discouraged, or in a lot of pain, or if labor has slowed. A change every 30 minutes or so may make a positive difference. During the birthing stage, too, the birthing person may use several different positions, especially if this stage takes more than an hour.

Just before the actual birth of the baby, the caregiver may ask the birthing person to assume a position where the caregiver feels more confident "catching the baby," such as semisitting or lying flat on their back with legs drawn up to the chest. Some caregivers, however, are comfortable with the birthing person in a variety of positions; see pages 171–176 for a list of useful positions and the possible benefits of each.

Most hospitals have birthing beds that can be raised or lowered and that have moving sections and add-ons that can be configured to support a birthing person in a variety of positions, such as semisitting, sitting upright, kneeling and leaning forward, and squatting with a bar for support. Most of these beds have electronic controls. When you first arrive at the hospital, push all the buttons to see how the bed works and try the many possible positions.

POSITIONS AND MOVEMENTS FOR LABOR AND BIRTH

STANDING

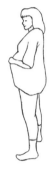

Unique Benefits:

- Takes advantage of gravity during and between contractions
- For some people in labor, it's more comfortable than sitting or lying down.
- Shortens contractions and helps them be more productive
- Helps position the fetus to enter the pelvis
- May speed labor if the laboring person has been lying down
- May increase the urge to push in the second stage

WALKING

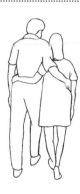

Unique Benefits:

- Same as standing, plus:
- Causes slight changes in the pelvic joints that encourage rotation and descent

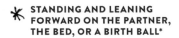

✱ STANDING AND LEANING FORWARD ON THE PARTNER, THE BED, OR A BIRTH BALL*

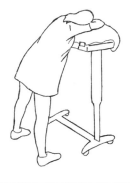

Unique Benefits:

- Same as standing, plus:
- Relieves backache
- Makes it easy for the partner or doula to give a back rub
- May be more restful than standing upright
- Can be used with an electronic fetal monitor (the laboring person must stand by the bed unless wireless monitors are used)

SLOW DANCING

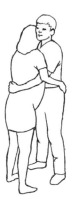

Movement:

The laboring person leans against the partner, resting their head on the partner's chest or shoulder. The partner's arms are around the laboring person, with fingers interlocked at their low back. The laboring person can tuck their thumbs into the partner's waistband or belt loops for comfort. They sway, perhaps to music, and breathe in rhythm.*

Unique Benefits:

- Same as standing, plus:
- Causes changes in the pelvic joints that encourage rotation and descent
- Being embraced by a loved one increases the laboring person's sense of well-being.
- Rhythm and music add comfort.
- Pressure from the partner's hands relieves back pain.

STANDING LUNGE

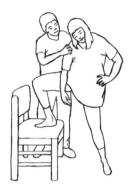

Movement:

Standing beside a chair and facing forward, the laboring person places one foot on the chair seat, with the raised knee and foot turned out. Bending the raised knee and hip, they "lunge" sideways repeatedly, slowly, and rhythmically during a contraction (either in the direction that is more comfortable, or to the right for two or three contractions and then to the left). They should feel the stretch in the inner thighs. Secure the chair and help keep them balanced.*

Unique Benefits:

- Widens the side of the pelvis toward which they lunge
- Gives room for the baby to change position if necessary
- May ease backache for a few contractions

KNEELING LUNGE

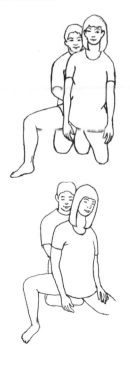

Movement:

From starting position: (a) slowly raise their knee and hip and "lunge" sideways, as in (b), and return to position (a) repeatedly during a contraction in the direction that is more comfortable, or if they feel the same, lunge to the right for 2 or 3 contractions and then to the left for 2 or 3. They should feel the stretch in the inner thighs.*

Unique Benefits:

- Same as standing lunge

* This positions are particularly helpful for slow labor or back labor.

SITTING UPRIGHT

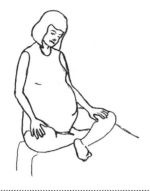

Unique Benefits:

- Gives the laboring person a rest between contractions
- Uses gravity to help the baby descend
- Can be used with an electronic fetal monitor

SITTING ON A TOILET OR COMMODE**

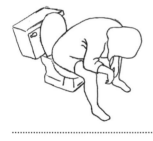

Unique Benefits:

- Same as sitting upright, plus:
- May help relax the perineum for effective bearing down

SEMISITTING**

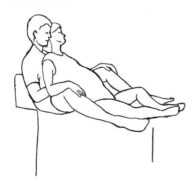

Unique Benefits:

- Same as sitting upright, plus:
- Makes a vaginal exam possible
- Easy position to get into on a bed or delivery table

SITTING AND ROCKING IN A CHAIR OR SWAYING ON A BIRTH BALL

Unique Benefits:

- Same as sitting upright, plus:
- May speed labor
- Helps relax the trunk and perineum

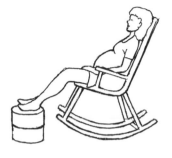

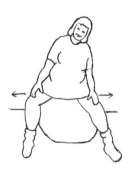

SITTING, LEANING FORWARD WITH SUPPORT*

Unique Benefits:

- Same as sitting upright, plus:
- Relieves backache
- Makes it easy for the partner to give a back rub

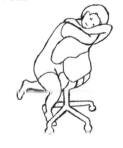

HANDS-AND-KNEES POSITION* **

Unique Benefits:

- Helps relieve backache
- Assists the rotation of a baby in OP position
- Allows for pelvic rocking and other body movements
- Takes pressure off hemorrhoids

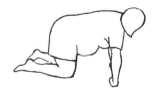

+ with rocking
+ with scarf looped under hips
to squeeze + lift hips

* These positions are particularly helpful for slow labor or back labor.
** These positions are also useful during the birthing stage.

KNEELING, LEANING FORWARD ON A CHAIR SEAT, THE RAISED HEAD OF THE BED, A BIRTH BALL, OR THE SIDE OF A TUB*

Unique Benefits:

- Same as hands and knees, plus:
- Puts less strain on wrists and hands
- Relieves back pain very effectively when done in a large tub

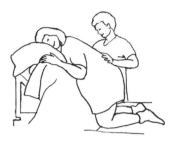

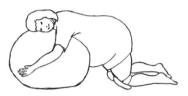

✳OPEN KNEE–CHEST POSITION

Movement:

Laboring person gets on hands and knees, lowers the chest, spreads the elbows, and rests their head on their hands. Make sure the knees are back far enough to raise the buttocks higher than the chest. You can support them by sitting on a chair, your feet about 9 inches (23 cm) apart. They put their head between your shins, and lean their shoulders against your shins.* This should be done for 30 to 45 minutes.

Unique Benefits:

- If partner's shins are uncomfortable, fold hand towels for padding.
- May be helpful in pre- or early labor
- Uses gravity to move baby's head (or buttocks) out of the pelvis, which may be desirable in early labor if the laboring person has backache or the baby is OP
- May reduce pressure on the cervix, which helps if it is swollen (also used for prolapsed cord; see page 131)

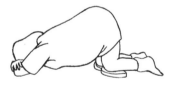

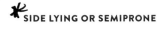 **SIDE LYING OR SEMIPRONE**

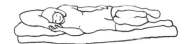

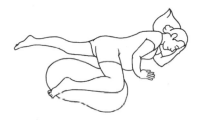

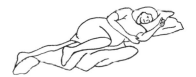

Movement:

In the side-lying position, the laboring person lies on their side with both knees flexed and a pillow between them (a). In the semiprone position, they straighten the lower leg, roll slightly toward the front, flex the top hip and knee, and rest the top knee on one or two pillows (b) or a peanut-shaped ball (c). During the birthing stage, you can hold the birthing person's top leg up as they push (d).**

Unique Benefits:

- Gives the laboring person some rest
- Makes interventions easy to perform
- Helps lower elevated blood pressure
- Safer than standing or the hands-and-knees position if pain medications are used
- May promote the progress of labor when alternated with walking
- Can slow a very rapid second stage
- Shifting between side-lying and semiprone positions helps change the baby's position.
- Works well with an epidural

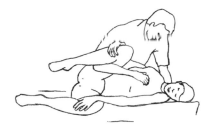

* These positions are particularly helpful for slow labor or back labor.

✳ SQUATTING

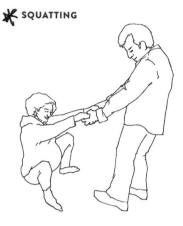

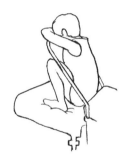

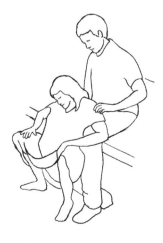

Movement:

The laboring person squats on the floor or bed, holding on to your hands (a) or a railing or a squatting bar (b) attached to the bed. Or, if you sit with your thighs spread, they may stand between your knees (facing away from you) and lower themselves into a squat, with their arms resting on your thighs for support (c).**

Unique Benefits:

- May relieve backache
- Uses gravity to help the baby descend
- May aid the baby's rotation
- Widens the pelvic outlet
- Provides the mechanical advantage of the upper trunk pressing on the uterus
- May help bring on the urge to push
- Requires less bearing-down effort
- Allows freedom to shift weight for comfort

LAP SQUATTING

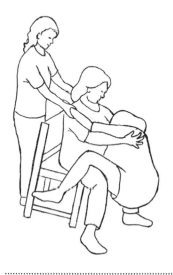

Movement:

Sit on an armless straight chair. The laboring person sits on your lap facing you, straddling your thighs. Embrace each other. When a contraction begins, spread your thighs, allowing their buttocks to sag between. Have a support person or doula stand behind you and hold the laboring person's hands for safety. After the contraction, bring your legs together and raise the laboring person onto your thighs again.**

CAUTION: This may not be possible if the laboring person weighs more than you can support.

Unique Benefits:

- Same as squatting, plus:
- Avoids strain on birthing person's knees and ankles
- Allows for more support with less effort for an exhausted laboring person
- Enhances feelings of well-being, as the laboring person is held close by a loved one

DANGLE WITH PARTNER

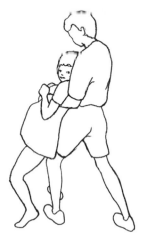

Movement:

Hold the laboring person under their arms as they lean with their back against you during contractions. They lower themselves so that you are bearing all their weight. Between contractions, they stand.**

Unique Benefits:

- Lengthens the laboring person's trunk, allowing more room for the baby to maneuver into position
- Enhances pelvic joint mobility, allowing the baby to push the pelvic bones as needed to descend
- Uses gravity to help the baby descend

CAUTION: This position requires much strength from the partner. See following for a way to dangle while the partner sits.

** These positions are also useful during the birthing stage.

DANGLE

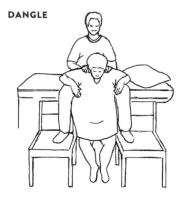

Movement:

Sit on the edge of a high bed or counter, with each foot supported on a chair and your thighs spread. Standing, the laboring person backs between your legs and places their flexed arms over your thighs. During contractions, they lower themselves as you grip their chest with your thighs. You support their full weight. Between contractions, they stand.**

Unique Benefits:

- Same as dangle with partner, plus:
- Puts much less strain on the partner

ON BACK WITH LEGS DRAWN UP

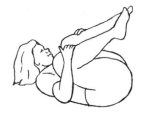

Movement:

The laboring person lies flat on their back, raises their chin, and holds their knees apart, drawing them to their shoulders. They lower their legs between contractions. You can help them get into position with each contraction.**

Unique Benefits:

- Do not use routinely
- Tiring and works against gravity
- May be helpful in prolonged second stage

✳ HANDS AND KNEES ROCKING FORWARD AND BACK

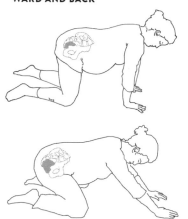

Movement:

The laboring person is on hands and knees (a); they rock back, flexing knees and hips (b). They may stay in position (b) or rock forward and back throughout the contraction.

Alternating positions (a) and (b) causes movement and changes shape of pelvic joints; position (b) increases dimensions of pelvic basin. It may aid fetal head rotation during second stage. (with thanks to Susan Steffes, P.T. for this suggestion)

** These positions are also useful during the birthing stage.

COMFORT AIDS AND DEVICES

In addition to the self-help comfort techniques you just learned about, there are also many comforting items or devices: some are built in or available in the birth setting; others you may wish to bring with you. Use the information here to explore these items and decide which you might want to use during labor. Most items are easily found in popular stores or online. If you cannot locate some, ask your childbirth educator, midwife, or doula where to get them.

Baths and Showers (Hydrotherapy)

One of the safest and most effective forms of pain relief in labor is immersion in deep water or a warm shower. Hydrotherapy has been used for relaxation, healing, and pain relief for centuries and today is widely used in physical therapy, sports medicine, and other health disciplines. Now, it is also widely used in childbirth. Showers are available in most hospitals, and bathtubs (some large enough for the laboring person to move around in or share with their partner) have been installed in many modern hospitals and birth centers. Some hospitals have tubs on wheels that can be moved from one birthing room to another. Lightweight tubs can be rented or purchased and set up temporarily in one's home for a home birth or possibly even in a hospital, if staff are willing and arrangements have been made in advance (see Recommended Resources, page 190).

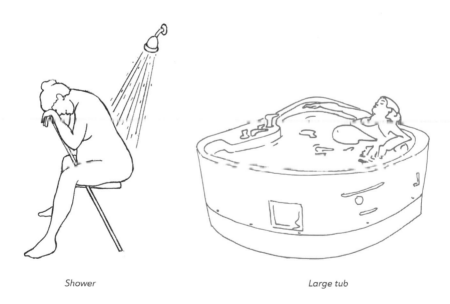

Shower

Large tub

✳ Try this fine?

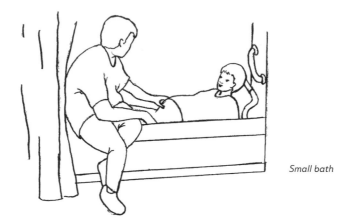

Small bath

Most people who use water in labor use it for pain relief. As you likely have experienced, soaking in a tub or lingering in the shower is soothing and relaxing. Numerous studies have shown that hydrotherapy, when used correctly during labor, is safe, reduces pain, and frequently speeds labor. It has advantages over pain medications: The laboring person can move about normally, and they remain clearheaded.

Showers and baths differ in their effects on the laboring person. While both enhance relaxation and reduce (but not eliminate) pain, the shower is simpler to use and requires fewer precautions. Water temperature is less of a safety concern with the shower than the bath (see page 79). The laboring person can use the shower early in labor, whereas the bath is better reserved until active labor. On the other hand, the shower is more tiring because one cannot easily recline, and it does not seem to have the labor-enhancing effects that immersion in deep water often has.

HOW DOES A BATH REDUCE PAIN AND SPEED ACTIVE LABOR?

When a laboring person sits in a deep, warm bath, a series of physiological changes begin immediately. These changes alter hormone production and fluid distribution throughout the body, quickly resulting in the following:

- Immediate relaxation and some pain relief from the warmth and buoyancy of the water, which can cause a drop in stress hormones
- Increasing oxytocin production in the pituitary gland, located in the brain, causing stronger contractions; labor progress often speeds up without an increase in pain.
- Feelings of calm and well-being, from the increased oxytocin (Note: intravenous oxytocin does not have calming effects because it does not reach the brain.)

These benefits last for up to 2 hours or so, after which changes in the laboring person's circulation often lead to a slowing of contractions. To prevent this, the laboring person might get out of the water after about 1½ hours or at any time the contractions seem to space out or become less intense. Once they have been out of the water for a 30 minutes or so, they can return.

WHEN SHOULD A LABORING PERSON GET INTO THE BATH?

As there is a time limit for benefits from the bath, the laboring person should not get in too early unless the caregiver wants to try to stop premature contractions or because they are having a long and tiring prelabor. Otherwise, the laboring person should wait until the cervix has dilated at least 5 centimeters and the contractions are clearly getting stronger and closer together (about 4 to 5 minutes apart), each lasting close to 1 minute. Getting into the bath at this point, they are likely to experience immediate and profound pain relief, along with faster dilation. Before this point they can take a long shower, which will not slow labor.

WHAT WATER TEMPERATURE IS BEST?

The water temperature should not be higher than body temperature—around 98.6°F (37°C). This is very important: If the water is too warm, the laboring person's temperature goes up, which can cause a fever in the baby. Even when it is not caused by infection, any rise in temperature can cause the baby's heart rate to increase too much for safety. The laboring person should get out and cool down; be sure the temperature of the water is correct before returning to the bath. Also, labor progress may slow if the water is too hot. And, if the laboring person feels uncomfortably hot, they may lose energy (and so will you if you are in the bath together!).

IS A BATH SAFE IF THE MEMBRANES HAVE RUPTURED?

Numerous research studies indicate that a bath in clean water does not increase the risk of infection if the person has ruptured membranes.

CAN STAFF MONITOR THE BABY WHILE THE PERSON LABORS IN THE WATER?

Yes. Most midwives who attend water births outside of hospitals have waterproof, hand-held ultrasound stethoscopes (Dopplers), and some hospitals also have these. A portable telemetry fetal-monitoring unit can be used as well.

There are two types of telemetry monitors. In one, a radio transmitter is wired to sensors on the laboring person's abdomen. As long as the radio is kept out of the water, it works well. In the other, which is wireless, each sensor contains its own waterproof transmitter. In both, the transmitters send information on the baby's heartbeat and the laboring person's contractions to the nursing station or to the monitor in the labor room.

WHAT IF THE BABY IS BORN IN THE WATER?

This is possible in a rapid labor, which is not always easy to control. If the hospital has a strong policy against birth in the water, the laboring person will need to be watched closely and will be asked to leave the bath when pushing begins. If born in the water, the baby is brought immediately to the surface and held with its head completely out of the water. The head is dried with a towel. The birthing person will be helped out of the water before the expulsion of the placenta.

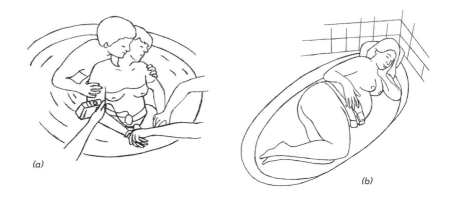

Laboring in a large bath with a partner (a) and using wireless telemetry fetal monitoring (b)

Water births are common and are considered a safe option for healthy pregnant people in hospitals in many countries, especially Europe and Australia. Numerous studies have found water birth to be as safe as birth on land when the caregiver is confident and skilled, the person is healthy, and labor has proceeded without complications. In North America, water births take place in homes, birth centers, and only a handful of hospitals. They are attended mostly by midwives, although a few doctors also attend water births (see Recommended Resources, page 190, for more information).

COMFORTING TECHNIQUES

In this section, we look at some simple techniques you can use to soothe and comfort the pregnant/laboring person, such as touch and massage, music, and pleasing scents. Practice them with the person and get their feedback to adapt them as needed.

Touch and Simple Massage

Touch conveys a kind, caring, comforting message to the laboring person. Find out what kind of touch the person finds soothing and use it during labor.

They may appreciate gentle, comforting, or reassuring touch— rubbing a painful spot, patting their back or shoulder, embracing them, holding their hand, scratching their back, or stroking their hair or cheek. With your fingertips or with your full hand, you might lightly stroke the skin on their abdomen during contractions, or the thighs, or wherever they want. Some people prefer a rhythmic rubbing or kneading of the back, legs, buttocks, shoulders, hands, or feet. (Because some laboring people find touch annoying, ask before doing it and check whether it is helping.)

Before beginning, pour a small amount of light massage oil into one palm and rub your hands together briskly to warm them and the oil. Some people like being rubbed or stroked during early labor but stop liking it during transition. If this happens, switch to holding the laboring person's head, shoulders, hand, foot, or thigh firmly, without rubbing. A massage device—handheld or battery-operated—may also be soothing and may be handy if you are not very good at massage.

HOW TO GIVE GREAT MINI-MASSAGES

During labor, brief, 1- to 3-minute, massages of the shoulders, back, hands, or feet may relax and soothe the laboring person. Practice these ahead of time to learn what they like. Perhaps they will even reciprocate! Follow these general guidelines:

- Explain which massage you want to do and ask permission ("I'd like to massage your back. Do you think that might feel good?").
- Make sure your hands are clean and warm and that the pregnant person is comfortable.
- Use massage oil—scented, if they like, although you'll want to have some unscented oil on hand for labor, in case anyone in the room is sensitive to scents. (Ask before using it.) Place a little oil on your hands and rub them together briskly to cover them with the oil and warm it.
- Once you begin the massage, try not to remove both hands at the same time. It is unsettling to relax into a massage only to have the massager's hands vanish without warning and to reappear somewhere else.
- As you work, encourage the pregnant person to tell you where they want more or less rubbing or a lighter or firmer touch.
- When you're finished, wipe any excess oil from their skin and your hands.

Following are some of my favorite mini-massages.

Three-part shoulder mini-massage: Use this massage during or between contractions, at any phase of labor, to help the laboring person feel nurtured and to relax their shoulders (shoulders are one of the most common tension spots in people). Have the laboring person sit up or lean forward and rest their head on their arms or a pillow. Stand behind them.

1. Place your hands comfortably on their shoulders near the neck. Stroke firmly from the neck to the shoulders and over the shoulders to their upper arms. Knead their upper arms a few times and stroke firmly back toward the neck. Do this three or four times.
2. With your hands on their shoulders, squeeze and release the shoulder muscles as firmly as they like for 1 to 2 minutes.

Crisscross massage over the small of the back and/or hips: Use this massage at any phase of labor, during or between contractions, to ease back pain or help relax the lower back.

Have the laboring person kneel and lean over the birth ball or a chair seat. It will be easiest for you if they use a ball on the bed, but you can also do this with them kneeling on the floor. They may want to wear kneepads or kneel on a foam pad such as those sold for gardeners.

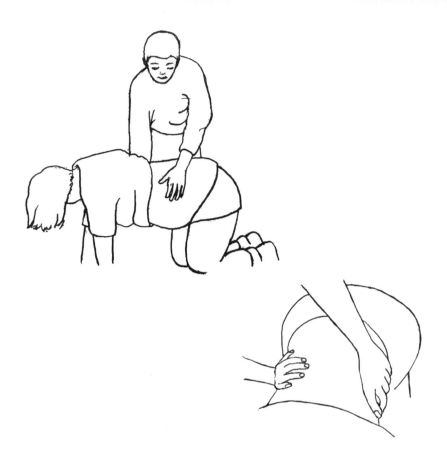

1. Facing the pregnant person's side, place your left hand on the narrowest part of their waist on the side farthest from you, with your fingers pointing down. Make sure your hands are not pressing on their ribs as that is uncomfortable. Place your right hand on their waist on the near side, fingers pointing up. Press their sides firmly; they should like the feeling. Keep your hands below their ribs and be sure you don't dig your fingertips into the soft flesh of their sides (it hurts!). If you have large hands, you may need to tilt them so they cover less surface area while staying within the small of their waist.

2. Using both hands, stroke firmly up, over, and across the back. (Cross one hand over the other to the original starting spots at their waist.)

3. Maintaining the same pressure, press the sides in again and repeat the crossover movement over and over as long as they want.

4. You may also move the crisscross strokes down over the hips and back up to the waist. Ask for feedback and adjust the placement and firmness as they wish.

"Breaking the ice pop" hand massage: If the laboring person has been clenching their fists or gripping your hand, the bedrail, or something else during contractions or if they seem generally tense, they are creating pressure on the palms of the hands where there are specialized nerve endings that are actually soothed by this pressure. Unfortunately, the gripping causes so much tension it loses much of its benefit. This quick massage technique will relax the hand and entire arm while providing the same pain-relieving pressure on the palm they were getting from gripping things. You can do this massage during or between contractions. Massage one hand, then the other, or have someone else do one hand while you do the other.

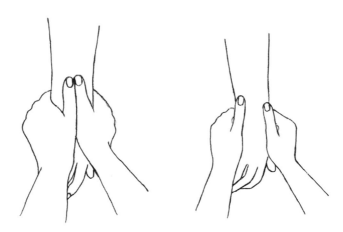

Thumbs together (left); thumbs apart (right) "breaking the ice pop" hand massage

1. Stand or sit facing the pregnant person. Ask them to relax their arm. Take their hand, palm down, in both of yours. Grasp the hand so your thumbs touch, from their tips to their fleshy bases, on the back of the wrist and the pads of your fingers (not your nails) press into the palm. Your thumb joints should be placed at their wrist joint (see illustration).
2. Without moving your hands, increase the pressure on the palm gradually. Ask for feedback so you know when you are squeezing "hard enough" for it to feel good. You may be surprised at how much pressure they like. When they say it is enough, maintain that pressure while slowly moving your thumbs and hands entirely off the back of their hand (see illustrations). You'll notice the skin on their hand blanches with your pressure. You are combining pressure on the palm with friction over the back of the hand. Adjust it so it feels good to them.

3. Repeat these strokes ten times or so. Does this massage remind you of how you broke apart twin ice pops when you were a child?

CAUTION: If the laboring person's hands are very swollen or if they have carpal tunnel syndrome (tingling or numbness in the hands that worsens with pressure), they will want very little pressure or not want this massage at all.

Three-part foot massage (breaking the ice pop with extras): If the laboring person complains of aching or tired feet during labor, this massage restores circulation and relieves tired aching feet caused by prolonged standing and walking.

1. Breaking the ice pop: Facing the pregnant person as they sit or lie down, ask them to relax their legs; take one foot in both your hands. Grasp it so your thumbs are together on the top of the foot. Press the pads of your fingers (not your nails) into the sole of the foot. Squeeze until the laboring person says it is enough. You may be surprised at how much pressure they like. Maintaining that pressure, move your thumbs and hands apart so your hands are entirely off the top of the foot. You are combining pressure on the sole of the foot with friction over the top of the foot. Do this ten times or so.

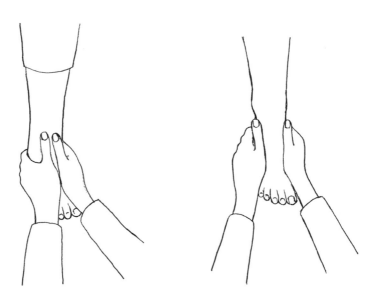

Part 1: Breaking the ice pop foot massage

2. Squeezing the heel: Cup the heel of the person's right foot in your right hand and press the "heel" of your hand firmly into the arch. Squeeze the person's heel firmly with the pads of your fingertips several times, as if you were squeezing a tennis ball, and release it. Avoid digging in with your nails. This should feel wonderful. Repeat, using your left hand to cup the person's left heel.

3. Three-finger circle massage: If you're massaging the left foot, hold it in your left hand; if you're working on the right foot, hold it in your right hand. With the pads of the three middle fingers of the opposite hand, give a deep circle massage in the "magic spot" on the top of the foot just below the ankle bone. The spot is slightly off the center of the foot, toward the outside. They'll tell you where it feels best. Do not move your fingers on the skin; rather, move the skin over the underlying muscles and bones. Do this for 30 to 60 seconds.

Once you have completed all three steps on one foot, repeat with the other foot. Then, they will be ready to walk some more!

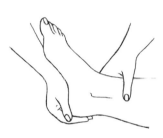

Part 2: Squeezing the heel: Press the "heel" of your hand into the arch of the person's foot; squeeze and release their heel.

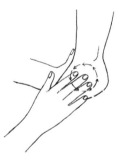

Part 3: Three-finger circle massage with fingertips

Music and Sound

Many people can relax and focus better if their favorite music, relaxation narration, or environmental sounds (ocean waves, a babbling brook, a rain shower) are played during labor. Familiar and well-loved music has been found to raise levels of endorphins (the body's own pain-relieving substances). Soothing sounds may cover up some of the beeps, voices, and other sounds that are part of any modern birthing room.

You might suggest that the pregnant person select some favorite music to play during labor. Make a playlist and bring your own player. Some laboring people appreciate having two labor playlists; one with calming, soothing music and a second with music that makes them want to get up and move.

CHAPTER 5

Strategies for Challenging Variations in Normal Labor

Labor, even when perfectly normal, rarely follows a predictable textbook pattern. Variations within a range of normal are to be expected. The emotional reactions of people in labor vary, depending on the type of labor pattern they have. For example, if prelabor or early labor drags on for a long time, both you and the laboring person may be challenged by exhaustion, worry, or a loss of confidence. If, instead, labor starts suddenly with long, painful contractions that threaten to overwhelm the laboring person, their pain and panic are the birth partner's main concerns. Laboring people and their birth partners cope best with labor when they are open and flexible and when they are confident they can and will (with the help of caregivers and a support team) handle whatever comes their way.

This chapter will help you deal with situations more stressful than those encountered in the average labor, but still falling within the range of "normal." These situations require more intense and active support from you. Both you and the laboring person will need more resourcefulness, effort, decision-making, patience, and reliance on the doula's or caregiver's encouragement and advice.

THE TAKE-CHARGE ROUTINE

When labor becomes very intense, the person in labor may feel panicked or frightened and may struggle to maintain rhythm or lose it entirely. If this happens, they need calm, confident, and kind, but firm, guidance to regain and maintain a rhythm. Reserve this routine for when the laboring person:

- Is unable to maintain a rhythmic ritual in breathing, moaning, or movements
- Despairs, weeps, cries out, or says they cannot go on
- Is very tense and cannot relax
- Is in a great deal of pain

The Take-Charge routine is exactly what it sounds like. You move in close and do all you can to help the person in labor until they regain their inner strength. Usually, their despair is brief; with your help, they can pass through it and their spirits will rise. If before labor they planned to request pain medication under these circumstances, use the Take-Charge routine to help until the medication can be given. Use whatever parts of this routine seem appropriate:

- Keep your touch firm and confident, not anxious and tense. Your voice should remain calm and encouraging. Your facial expression should reflect confidence and optimism.
- Stay close. Face the person in labor or stay right by their side, your face near theirs.
- Anchor them. Hold their shoulders or hands—gently, confidently, firmly. Do not shake them to get their attention.
- Get the laboring person to look at you. If their eyes are clenched shut, you will not be able to help. Tell them to open their eyes and look at your face or your hand. This is important. Say it loudly enough so they hear you—but calmly and kindly.
- Talk to them between contractions. Make suggestions; for example, "With the next one, let me help you more. I want you to look at me the moment it starts. I will pace you with my hand so it won't get ahead of us. Okay? Good. You're doing so well. We're really moving now."
- Help them regain the rhythm they had by moving your hand or head up and down in that rhythm. You can combine this with "rhythm talk" (see next item). Pause briefly after each downbeat to keep from going too fast.

One doula said, "I wear a ring with a blue stone on my right hand. I ask the laboring person to "follow my ring" as I "conduct" them in a breathing rhythm. I love to think of the many, many women who have let my ring guide them through some tough moments. It's one reason I never take the ring off."

- Use "rhythm talk, vocally pacing the rhythm of their breathing or moaning. Say, "Breathe with me ... BREATHE WITH ME ... That's the way ... just like that ... Good ... Keep your rhythm ... STAY WITH IT ... just like that ... LOOK AT ME ... Keep your rhythm ... Good for you ... It's going away ... Good ... Good ... Now just rest, that was so good."

You can whisper these words or say them in a calm, rhythmic, confident, and encouraging tone. If the laboring person is vocalizing, you may have to raise your voice to get their attention, but do not shout. Also, you don't actually need to breathe with the person as you say the words; you shouldn't even try if your breath is stale or the breathing makes you lightheaded. They can breathe to the rhythm of your words as well as your hand or head movements.

- Repeat yourself. The laboring person may not be able to continue doing what you say for more than a few seconds, but that's fine. Do not conclude that what you are doing is not helping. Say the same things repeatedly and help them continue.

What if the laboring person says they can't or won't go on? Here are some guidelines:

- Between contractions, tell them you want them to change the ritual used during contractions because it is no longer working. Suggest a different position or breathing rhythm.
- Don't give up on them. This is a difficult time. You cannot help if you decide they cannot handle it. Acknowledge to both the laboring person and to yourself that it is difficult, but remind yourselves it is not impossible.
- Ask for help and reassurance. It can be very hard on you to see the person you love in pain. The nurse or caregiver can check the laboring person's dilation and give you advice. Perhaps the person in labor is in distress because labor is progressing very rapidly; just knowing this may help. A doula or other support person can help you, model the technique for you, suggest something new, and reassure both of you that the laboring person is okay and reacting normally. If you're having trouble with the Take-Charge routine, the doula might "take charge" while you hold the laboring person or press on their back.
- Remember the baby. It may seem surprising, but laboring people can get so caught up in labor they do not think much about the baby. It may help to remember why they are going through this and to recognize that the baby is working with them.
  What about **pain medications**? Should you suggest them or not? This depends on:
- The laboring person's prior wishes: Did they want a nonmedicated birth? How strongly did they feel about it? (See "Pain Medications Preference Scale," pages 145–146.) Sometimes, people who ask for pain medications are really saying, "I need more help coping."
- Their rate of progress and how far they still have to go. A couple centimeters (1 inch) of dilation should be very encouraging. A complete lack of progress is very discouraging.
- How well they respond to the Take-Charge routine or the doula's help. If the person in labor cannot get back into a rhythm, even with a lot of help, and they are making little progress, they may need pain medications.
- Whether they are willing to try something else, such as a bath, a change of position, a progress check, or just coping with three more contractions to see whether things get easier
- Whether they truly want the medications or are just agreeing to the nurse's or caregiver's suggestion
- Whether they ask for medications between contractions. Many people ask for medications during a contraction, but do not mention them when the contraction ends.
- Whether they use the code word (see page 147)

Numerous people have said to their partners, "I never could have done it without you. If it hadn't been for you, I would have given up." By using the Take-Charge routine, you can indeed get the laboring person through those desperate moments when they feel they cannot go on; you can truly ease their burden by helping them with every breath. And if you both agree in advance on a code word they can use if they decide they want medications, you will know you're not forcing them to suffer.

THE VERY RAPID LABOR

For some people, labor starts with intense, frequent, painful contractions and is over in a matter of a few hours. It seems the laboring person barely has time to adjust to being in labor before the baby is born.

Sometimes, only the first (dilation) stage is rapid. The cervix dilates so quickly that the laboring person can't catch up mentally; but then, in the second (birthing) stage, the contractions space out. If this happens, the laboring person has to cope with the difficulties of both fast and slow labors.

It is impossible to predict which people will labor in these ways, but a rapid labor seems to be more likely if:

- The pregnant person has had a rapid or quicker-than-average (less than 10-hour) labor before. A second or third labor tends to be faster than the first.
- The cervix is very soft, thin, and already partially dilated before labor begins, and the baby is low in the pregnant person's pelvis in a very favorable position.
- The bag of waters ruptures with a gush rather than a slow leak, especially if accompanied by contractions.

Few people or their birth partners are prepared for a rapid labor, especially after reading and hearing about typical labor patterns and prolonged prelabors. The pregnant person will be caught off guard if expecting that early contractions will be gentle, short, and far apart, but instead has contractions that are long, painful, and close together—almost like the contractions of the transition phase.

How Is the Laboring Person Likely to React?

You can expect any of the following reactions from the laboring person if labor begins rapidly:

- Shock and disbelief. They may not be able to respond constructively or even realize this is real labor.
- Fear or panic. They may think something is terribly wrong—that they or the baby is in danger. They may be frightened if they cannot reach you, the caregiver, or anyone else for help and may worry about getting to the hospital in time. Make alternative plans for these possibilities. Make sure you are always reachable by phone, AND have a Plan B— a friend, neighbor, or family member who agrees to be reachable (and whom you keep informed of times when you may not be immediately available). The pregnant person can call a cab or a car service (be sure you have saved numbers and a way to pay). Plan C is to call 911 and say they are in hard labor and have no way to get to the hospital.
- Loss of confidence. If the laboring person thinks these are the "easy" contractions of early labor, they may lose all confidence in the ability to cope with labor once it progresses.
- Dependence on you. They may barely be able to change positions between contractions, let alone get ready to go to the hospital. They may need your constant help to cope with the contractions.

- Annoyance with you or the caregivers if neither of you grasps the situation. (People tell stories of their partners going back to sleep, assuming there is a long wait ahead, and of caregivers who tell them to go to sleep, which is impossible, or to wait an hour and then call again.)

How Should You React?
- Believe what you see. If the laboring person is shaky, in pain, and having strong, fast contractions, don't assume they are overreacting to early labor. Assume this is hard labor and move right into a leadership role to help them cope.
- Don't worry about helping them relax. These contractions will not allow that.
- Use the Take-Charge routine (see page 86) if they have trouble coping with the contractions.
- Don't lose faith in them or criticize them. Give them the benefit of the doubt. Their response is telling you this labor is really hard.
- Call the caregiver, go to the hospital or birth center, or both. Drive carefully, but don't waste time.

WHEN LABOR MUST START (LABOR-STIMULATING MEASURES)

Under some circumstances, the caregiver recognizes that delaying or awaiting the baby's birth for much longer carries unacceptable risks for the pregnant person or baby. The caregiver will suggest labor induction—starting labor by giving drugs, breaking the bag of waters, or other means (see "Induction or Augmentation of Labor," page 114). Rarely, the caregiver may believe that a medical induction should be done immediately (see page 115), but more often, the need is not urgent and you and the pregnant person may have a few days to try self-induction methods. If successful, they can avoid medical induction, which carries some risks and challenges (see disadvantages of induction for medical reasons, page 115).

Many doctors offer induction routinely at 39, 40, or 41 weeks, for no medical reason. This is called elective induction; see pages 114–118 for a discussion of medical and non-medical reasons for induction and use the Key Questions for Informed Decision-Making (see page 101) to recognize whether induction is medically indicated or not. It is usually safer, especially for the first-time birthing person, to wait for labor to begin spontaneously than to have an elective medical induction or to try self-induction.

Why try self-induction methods? Probably the most compelling reason is that medical induction is considered to be indicated if the pregnant person goes two weeks beyond the due date. If they wish to avoid a medical induction and is at 41½ weeks, they may want to try to get labor to begin. Another reason could be a steadily rising blood pressure or that the baby's growth has slowed, in which case the doctor may advise induction in a few days.

Self-induction may or may not succeed. If it does not succeed, the pregnant person will end up with a medical induction anyway. Some people feel it is worth trying to get into labor on their own; others do not. The methods are easy to use and carry little risk, which persuades some to try them (but see the following sections for precautions). Chances of success depend on the pregnant person's readiness for labor (the cervix must be ripe and have begun to thin) and the techniques chosen.

SELF-INDUCTION METHODS

Before using these techniques to start labor, make sure the pregnant person discusses them with the caregiver. Consult the caregiver as to whether there is any reason they should not try to start contractions, using the methods described here. If there are none, it is safe for you both to get started.

Nipple Stimulation

Stimulating the pregnant person's nipples causes the release of oxytocin, a hormone that contracts the uterus. Taking advantage of this physiological connection between breast and uterus may start labor or at least cause some contractions. Nipple stimulation probably will not work, however, if the cervix has not ripened or thinned significantly or if the pregnant person is currently breastfeeding a toddler, in which case their body has adapted to increased levels of oxytocin. The caregiver can tell them how ready the cervix is after a vaginal exam.

Either you or the pregnant person can stimulate the nipples, in one or more of the following ways, to bring on or intensify contractions:

- Lightly stroke, roll, or brush one or both nipples with the fingertips. Or, you can caress, lick, or suck the nipples. Often, within a few minutes the pregnant person will have strong contractions. The stimulation may need to be kept up intermittently for hours to keep the contractions coming.
- Massage the breasts gently with warm, moist towels for an hour at a time, three times a day.
- Use a gentle but powerful electric breast pump with double-pumping capability (which allows you to pump both breasts at once). A manual or battery-operated breast pump is less likely to work as well as one with a wall plug. Pump one breast for 30 minutes, three to five times per day, pausing when a contraction begins and resuming when it stops.

Start with one nipple or one breast. If stimulating only one does not initiate contractions in a reasonable length of time or if the contractions already occurring do not increase in frequency, length, or strength, try stimulating both breasts at once, between contractions at first, and then, if necessary, continuously. If there are no contractions after 1 to 2 hours, wait a half day before trying again or try some of the other methods.

PRECAUTIONS WHEN USING NIPPLE STIMULATION.

Many caregivers are very comfortable with their clients' use of nipple stimulation to bring on labor; others are wary because stimulating the nipples sometimes causes excessively long or strong contractions. These caregivers worry that strong contractions may stress the fetus, especially if the pregnant person is at high risk for complications. Before approving the use of nipple stimulation, the caregiver may want to check the baby's response to such stimulation by trying nipple stimulation first during electronic fetal monitoring in the hospital or office.

To help avoid excessively strong or long contractions, it is wise to time the length and assess the intensity of all contractions resulting from nipple stimulation. Stop stimulating the breasts if contractions become painful or long (more than 60 seconds).

Walking

Although effective in speeding a slow labor, walking is unlikely to get labor started. If you both want to try it anyway, take a fairly brisk walk, but don't go too far from home or the labor room. If nothing else, walking is a pleasant distraction before labor.

Sexual Stimulation

Sexual intercourse with orgasm is the most effective form of sexual stimulation in starting labor. Orgasm causes the release of oxytocin and contractions of the uterus, and it may also cause the release of prostaglandins, hormone-like substances that soften the cervix. Semen also contains prostaglandins.

Clitoral stimulation by hand or mouth, even without orgasm or intercourse, may also be effective in bringing on contractions.

If you choose one of these methods, make them as pleasant as possible. Try to forget your goal of starting labor and free yourselves to enjoy the sexual experience—more than once, if needed. Frequent intercourse or clitoral stimulation—several times a day—may be needed to get into labor.

PRECAUTIONS WHEN USING SEXUAL STIMULATION

- Avoid placing anything within the vagina if the membranes have ruptured because doing so increases the risk of infection.
- Do not blow into the vagina.
- Avoid these methods if either of you has any sores that could spread or if the pregnant person has an uncomfortable vaginal condition.

THE SLOW-TO-START LABOR

Another challenging type of labor is the one that is slow to start. In this case, contractions, sometimes painful, go on for hours or days before the cervix finally begins to dilate. We don't know exactly why this happens to some but not to others, but if the following conditions are present, it might be more likely they will have a slow-to-start labor:

- The cervix is still long (or thick), firm, and posterior when contractions begin (see "Labor Progresses in Six Ways," page 24).
- The cervix is scarred from previous surgery or injury. A scarred cervix may resist thinning and so may require more time and more intense contractions to overcome this resistance. Once thinning occurs, labor usually progresses normally.

- The uterus is contracting in an uncoordinated fashion so the contractions do not open the cervix. The reason for this is not understood, but the condition often resolves with time, rest, or medications to promote sleep or induce labor (see page 114).
- The baby's head is high in the pelvis (see page 19) or in an unfavorable position, such as OP (occiput posterior; see page 19), or other presentations, such as face, brow, or head tilted toward one shoulder (called asynclitism). Some babies have a hand up by their face.
- The pregnant person is very anxious and tense about labor or the baby. Increased production of stress hormones (such as adrenaline) in early labor can interfere with labor progress.

Most slow-to-start labors eventually hit their stride with time and strong contractions and proceed normally after the initial long prelabor period. Some slow-to-start labors, however, are part of a generally prolonged labor, in which all phases proceed, but at a very slow pace. When a labor begins slowly, you cannot know in advance just when it will speed up—only time will tell. Fatigue and discouragement can present a serious challenge in this type of labor, and medical interventions may be required. Your role as birth partner will be to maintain the laboring person's morale and help them pace themselves mentally and physically. If interventions are being considered by the caregiver, you can also help the laboring person be well informed about the options (see pages 101).

Strategies for a Slow-to-Start Labor

If the laboring person's long prelabor is tiring and discouraging, though not necessarily painful, the following measures will help:

- Be patient and confident. This labor will not go on forever, and your positive attitude will help keep their spirits up.
- If the laboring person is worried, remind them that a long prelabor does not necessarily mean something is wrong with them or the baby. The cervix simply needs more time before it thins and begins opening. The two of you need to find ways to wait without worrying.
- Call friends, family, the caregiver, or your doula for encouragement and morale boosting. Do not call anyone who will make you worry more. A doula, with their confidence, experience, and perspective, can be a great help in such labors. One doula, attending a slow-to-start labor, and, to get the parents' minds off the slow progress, suggested they all read a play together. The only play they had was Shakespeare's The Tempest—not an easy play to read! But the mother read her parts, and it worked as a good distraction. Before long, her labor had picked up!
- Try not to become preoccupied with the labor, analyze, or overreact to every contraction. This will only make the labor seem longer.
- Encourage the pregnant person to eat and drink high-carbohydrate, easily digested foods (for example, toast with jam, cereals, pancakes, pasta, fruit juice, coconut water, tea with sugar or honey, sorbet, or gelatin desserts).

- Create a clean, tidy environment with whatever makes the pregnant person comfortable—music, a fire in the fireplace, flowers, favorite scents, and so on.

Additionally, you can help pass the time by rotating among distracting, restful, and labor-stimulating activities. Here are some suggestions:

1. During the day, try distracting activities. Encourage the pregnant person to get out of the house. If they are willing and up to it, visit friends, go for a walk, get a massage, go to work or go to a movie, the mall, or a restaurant (you can hope you'll have to leave before you finish your meal!). You'll find that when out of the house, they will try to minimize their reactions to the contractions and, thus, avoid overreacting to them. This is easier to do when they're among other people than when alone at home.

2. At home, you can utilize these distracting activities: dance; clean; pay bills; play games; start a project such as baking bread, cookies, or a birthday cake (they might almost hope that labor doesn't start until the project is finished!); wash and put away the baby's clothes; arrange or file photos; fix and freeze meals for after the baby is born; have friends over, especially to relieve you if you are tired.

3. Help the pregnant person rest or sleep at night or nap during the day. If they are tired but cannot sleep, try the following:
   - A bath: Fill the tub with warm (not hot) water; provide an inflatable bathtub pillow or folded towels for a headrest. They should plan to stay in the tub for a long time; you may have to add hot water from time to time to keep it warm enough. Rest and sleep may come more easily in a warm bath. Keep an eye on them; make sure they don't slip down with their head under the water. Remember, a bath tends to slow contractions in early labor and should be used only when the laboring person needs a rest.
   - If a bath is not an option, encourage a long, warm shower. You might need to turn up the water heater.

CAUTION ABOUT BATHS: A deep, warm bath can slow contractions, but there may be circumstances when slowing labor is not appropriate—e.g., they are overdue; the bag of waters has broken and an induction may be done if labor does not pick up on its own; or other reasons.

Also, be careful not to exceed a water temperature of about 98°F (37°C), as the laboring person may become overheated (see page 79 for more information), which can slow labor when it is still early.

- Play soothing music.
- Give a back rub.
- Offer a relaxing beverage (warm milk, herbal tea).
- Use relaxation techniques and slow breathing during contractions (see page 61). Try labor-stimulating measures for periods of 1 to 2 hours at a time to initiate stronger, more frequent contractions. Follow the guidelines in "When Labor Must Start," page 90, noting the precautions for these procedures.

4. If the pregnant person is not only sleepless but also in pain, long baths, relaxation, massage, and slow breathing will help. See "Self-Help Comfort Measures," page 58, for ideas.

5. Try different positions and movements. The following positions and movements sometimes stimulate labor, by taking advantage of gravity, changing the shape of the laboring person's pelvis, or encouraging the baby to wiggle into a better position, while relieving backache.
   - Open knee–chest position (see page 72)
   - Hands and knees, with or without pelvic rocking (see page 172)
   - Walking and slow dancing (see pages 67 and 68)

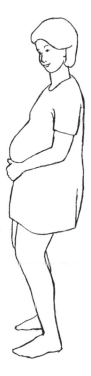 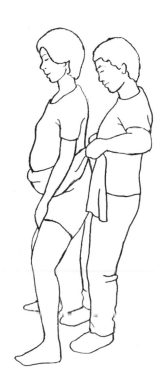

   - Abdominal lifting: While standing, the pregnant person interlocks their fingers and places them against the pubic bone under the pregnant belly. During contractions, they lift the abdomen up and slightly in, while bending their knees. This often relieves back pain while improving the position of a baby in the pelvis. You can help them by standing behind them, placing a long woven shawl, folded to about 5 inches (13 cm) wide, around their trunk and below the abdomen, and lifting the abdomen as shown in the illustration. Loosen it when the contraction is over.

CAUTION: Rarely, the abdominal lift makes the baby uncomfortable, causing the baby to wiggle more, indicating it's uncomfortable—so stop doing it. If you have a nurse or midwife with you, it is a good idea to ask them to listen to the baby's heartbeat during a contraction while doing the abdominal lift. These precautions are taken because it is possible, though very rare, that the umbilical cord could be in a place where it can be pressed by the shawl. If so, the abdominal lift should not be done.

The laboring person can alternate these positions and movements with rest.

If these strategies are not enough to get them through a long prelabor, the caregiver may suggest an alcoholic beverage, morphine, sleep medication, or another drug.

If the two of you are worried that the pregnant person won't have the stamina to cope with "real" labor after this prolonged prelabor, remind yourself—and them—that they are well equipped at this time in their life to cope with a long period without sleep. Although they feel tired and discouraged, once labor begins to make progress, their energy level and spirits will likely rise, allowing them to continue without distress. If not, they may benefit from pain medications that allow them to rest.

SLOW PROGRESS IN ACTIVE LABOR AND THE BIRTHING STAGE—WITH OR WITHOUT BACK PAIN

Sometimes, labor begins with good progress but it slows once the person gets into active labor (after 5 or 6 centimeters). We usually expect progress to speed up around this time. The delay may be temporary, or progress may continue to be slow until the birth. This delay is sometimes associated with back pain, sometimes not.

One in three people have back pain during active labor—or back labor. One possible cause is a poor fit between the baby's head and the pregnant person's pelvis. The actual size of the baby's head is less often a problem than its position in the pelvis. The most favorable head position is occiput anterior, or OA (where the back of the baby's head is toward the pregnant person's front), with the baby's chin tucked to their chest. When, instead, the back of the baby's head is toward the pregnant person's back (OP, occiput posterior), or is tightly positioned sideways (OT, occiput transverse), or tipped back or to one side, then a larger diameter of the baby's head is pressing down into the pelvis. If the baby's hand is placed next to their face as they enter the pelvis, it can also cause back pain and so can variations in the pregnant person's pelvic and spinal anatomy. All these factors, and others, may cause a delay in labor as well as back pain. Reducing this pain and repositioning the baby are the major goals when supporting the laboring person.

As for comfort measures for backache during labor, relaxation and breathing are usually not enough to cope with the pain. Try one or more of the following comfort measures, described in chapter 4: counter- pressure, crisscross massage, the double hip squeeze, rolling pressure over the low back, heat and cold, baths and showers, and transcutaneous electrical nerve stimulation (TENS).

Problems that cause both back pain and a delay in active labor usually resolve spontaneously, but this is likely to happen more quickly if the laboring person is active and trying ways to help the baby change position.

Encouraging the Baby to Change Position

It is not always easy to identify the baby's position in the pelvis; even the most experienced nurses, midwives, and doctors have trouble doing this sometimes. However, you do not need to know the baby's position before trying some of the measures described in this and the preceding chapter.

If there is a delay in active labor, whether or not the laboring person has back pain, assume there is a need to change the baby's position.

Help the laboring person use the following positions and movements to encourage the baby to change position. Some of these techniques may also relieve back pain:

- Pelvic rocking (see page 76)
- Slow dancing (see page 68)
- Abdominal lifting (see page 95)
- The lunge (see page 69), during contractions. Have them lunge, using rhythmic patterns, in each direction and then continue with the most comfortable direction for five or six contractions. Help them keep their balance and keep the chair from sliding. The lunge is not easy to do, but it may very well correct the problem.
- Side lying, where the laboring person lies on their side with both hips and knees flexed and a pillow between the knees. If the nurse or midwife is quite sure the baby's back is toward the left side of the laboring person's back (left occiput posterior, or LOP), they lay on their left side; if they believes the baby is ROP, the laboring person lies on the right side. If you are not sure of the baby's position, have them turn from one side to the other every 20 to 30 minutes.

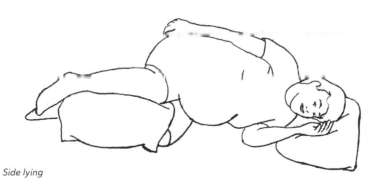

Side lying

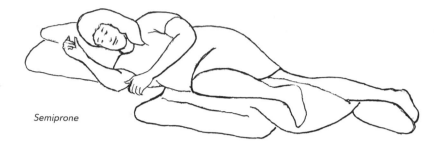

Semiprone

- Lying semiprone: If the nurse or midwife thinks the baby's back is toward the left side of the birthing person's back (LOP), they lie in the right semiprone position—on their right side with the lower leg out straight. The upper hip and knee are flexed, resting the upper knee on a doubled-up pillow or peanut-shaped ball, and they roll toward their front.

  If the baby's back is toward the right side of their back, they lie the same way on their left side. Unless you are sure of the baby's position, have the birthing person change sides every 20 to 30 minutes.

Note: The semiprone position is quite different in its gravity effects than the side-lying position, so instructions regarding which side to lie on are different for the two positions.

- Kneeling and leaning forward: The birthing person rests their upper body on a chair or a birth ball. Some special hospital beds, called birthing beds, can be adjusted to support this position.
- Standing and walking: These take advantage of gravity in encouraging the baby to descend. In addition, the alignment of the baby within the pelvis is thought to be most favorable when the birthing person is upright. Walking also allows some movement within the pelvic joints, which may encourage the baby's rotation.

Promoting the Baby's Descent in the Birthing Stage

If there is a delay in descent during the birthing stage, it is important that the birthing person change position. They can try shifting from semisitting to side lying to squatting to sitting on the toilet. They can try unconventional positions such as the dangle, lap squatting, and lying on their back while lifting their head and drawing their knees up toward their armpits. All these positions are described and illustrated on pages 67–76.

Note: The positions that require getting out of bed are next to impossible if the birthing person has been given an epidural (see pages 70–73 for positions to use with an epidural).

Also, the dangle and lap squatting require practice ahead of time and may not be acceptable to the hospital staff. If you think these positions are ones you both might want to try, discuss this with the caregiver ahead of time. Also rehearse them ahead of time to be sure you are comfortable with them.

Occasionally, a baby will not reposition, despite the birthing person's efforts—especially if the baby is large. If so, the baby may be born facing forward ("sunny-side up"). Otherwise, medical or surgical interventions are likely needed to deliver the baby. Possibilities include pain medications (usually an epidural); intravenous oxytocin to strengthen the contractions (see page 115); delivery with forceps or a vacuum extractor (see pages 120–122); or, if nothing else works, a cesarean delivery (see pages 147–157). It's wise to read about these procedures ahead of time.

You can help the birthing person deal with a delay in labor by:

- Being very empathetic
- Maintaining patience and optimism
- Helping them change position so the baby can change position and descend
- Using the techniques described in chapter 4 to relieve any back pain
- Ask the Key Questions for Informed Decision-Making (see page 101)

The caregiver's role in this situation is described on pages 129–133 in chapter 7.

WHEN THE BIRTHING PERSON MUST LABOR IN BED

Sometimes, a person must remain in bed for labor and birth. These are the most common reasons:

- High blood pressure: One's high blood pressure tends to drop when lying on the left side.
- Pain medications: If one is sleepy or groggy or if half the body is numb with an epidural, they are able to move in bed but cannot safely get out of bed.
- Use of equipment that attaches to machines: Intravenous lines, electronic fetal monitors, bladder catheters (thin tubes), and other devices all tend to make it difficult or impossible to move out of bed.
- Hospital customs: Unfortunately, in many hospitals, even people with normal labors are routinely discouraged from leaving their beds. There is no medical reason for such a practice.

Being restricted to bed may not distress the birthing person, especially if they are tired, are comfortable in bed, or this was expected. Some, though, find that lying down is most uncomfortable in labor. Some become very restless and are unable to stay down. A person who planned to use movement and positioning for comfort or to help the labor progress will be disappointed and should ask to get out of bed.

Sometimes, restricting a person to bed slows the labor and increases the pain from contractions. It also prevents the laboring person from doing many of the things that speed labor and increase comfort.

Here are some things you can do if the laboring person does not have an epidural and is confined to bed:

1. Find out the reason: The two of you may be able to persuade the caregiver to change the orders if there is no compelling medical reason to remain in bed. If bed rest is medically necessary, you will both be better able to accept it and cooperate if you understand the reason.

2. Find out how strict the order is: The laboring person may be told not to leave the bed or not to turn from their left side at all. They may be allowed up for short periods or to go to the bathroom or to take a bath, which could be as effective for lowering blood pressure as lying on the left side. These options make a positive difference.

3. Ask about alternatives: The laboring person may be able to use a telemetry unit (see page 108) for electronic fetal monitoring and an IV pole on wheels. These allow getting out of bed and walking. Even if connected to many machines and containers, they may be able to stand or to sit in a rocker beside the bed.

4. Help the laboring person focus on the many pain-coping techniques and comfort measures that can be used while in bed, without dwelling too much on what cannot be done. Try relaxation (see page 58), rhythmic breathing (see page 61), attention focusing (see page 59), spontaneous rituals (see page 151), massage (see pages 80–85), transcutaneous electrical nerve stimulation (TENS; see page 194), hypnosis (learned ahead of time, see page 193), or the Take-Charge routine (see page 86).

Although remaining in bed may add to the laboring person's stress, with your help, they can handle this challenge. The key is to understand and accept the reasons for remaining in bed, to focus on the comfort techniques that can be used, and not to give up.

CHAPTER 6

Tests, Technologies, Interventions, and Procedures

THE CAREGIVER'S PRIMARY ROLE IN CHILDBIRTH is to safeguard the health of the laboring person and baby. Throughout pregnancy, the caregiver relies on a wide assortment of tests, technologies, and procedures to detect and treat problems before they become serious. Similar tests, technologies, and procedures (often referred to as "interventions") are available during childbirth.

Caregivers differ regarding what constitutes routine basic care during childbirth. Some caregivers feel birth is so unpredictable it is safest to use many medical procedures in every labor, whether needed or not. Others believe childbirth is essentially a normal physiological process and use medical or surgical interventions only when problems are suspected or detected. Pregnant people differ over the same issues. Some are fearful and feel more secure with a highly medical approach, while others perceive birth as normal and are wary of excessive interventions. They place more trust in their bodies and inner resources than in technology.

Research has shown that, for a healthy person, labor proceeds normally and safely most of the time and that careful observation is all that is necessary to detect problems in time to take medical action.

One way to *avoid* problems is to be cautious about using optional procedures and medications; these can sometimes *cause* problems. For example, any procedure that restricts the laboring person's freedom to move might slow labor or increase pain, thus making further interventions more likely and increasing the risk of developing other problems. For these reasons, technology, medications, and procedures are appropriate and necessary only when problems already exist or are very likely to occur.

KEY QUESTIONS FOR INFORMED DECISION-MAKING

Tests and interventions always involve tradeoffs. The laboring person needs to know what they give up and what they gain before deciding whether to accept a nonemergency intervention. When considering interventions, discuss the following questions with each other and with the caregiver.

When a test is suggested, ask:

- What is the reason for the test?
- What questions will it answer?
- How is the test done?
- How accurate or reliable are the results? What is the margin of error? In other words, might the test miss a problem that exists or indicate a problem that does not exist?
- If the test detects a problem, what happens next (for example, further testing or immediate treatment)?
- If the test does not detect a problem, what happens next (for example, a repeat test in a day or two, other tests, or no further concern about the problem)?
- What will this test cost the pregnant person, if anything?

When a treatment or intervention is suggested, ask:

- What is the problem and how serious is it?
- How urgent is the need to begin treatment?
- What is the treatment and how is it done?
- How likely is it to solve the problem?
- If the treatment fails, what are the next steps?
- Are there any side effects to the treatment?
- Are there any alternatives (including waiting, doing nothing, or other treatments)?

If an alternative is suggested, again, ask how it is done, how likely it is to work, what its side effects are, and what happens if the alternative treatment fails.

In most situations, there is plenty of time to discuss these questions. When you, the pregnant person, and your caregiver exchange information, questions, and concerns and come to a decision together, it is called "shared decision-making." This approach builds trust and satisfaction because it is based on mutual respect, flexibility, and consideration for each other's points of view.

In the rare case of a true emergency, however, there may not be time for such discussion. The caregiver should tell you how serious and urgent the situation is. If it is urgent, you must trust the caregiver and help the laboring person accept the interventions. A full explanation may have to wait until the emergency is over. In this case, simply ask, "Will this intervention improve the odds of a healthy birthing parent and healthy baby?" If the answer is yes, agree to it, no questions asked. Explanations and discussion may have to come later.

During the last month of pregnancy, pregnant people usually see their caregivers once a week. This is a time when problems that can affect labor may surface for the first time, and their detection now, may help the caregiver plan how best to care for the laboring person during labor. Following are descriptions of some common late-pregnancy tests and why and how they are done. This information cannot substitute for discussing the key questions (see page 101) with the caregiver but may provide background on which to base your questions. Omitted here are routine tests given in early pregnancy or at every prenatal checkup.

LATE-PREGNANCY TESTS

During the final weeks or months of pregnancy, the caregiver watches closely for conditions in either the pregnant person or the baby that might affect the outcome of the birth. Results of the tests described here guide the caregiver in planning the clinical management of the birth.

Group B Strep (GBS) Screening

This tests the pregnant person for the presence of particular bacteria, called Group B streptococci. Offered at 35 to 37 weeks of pregnancy, the test involves culturing a sample of secretions from the vagina and/or rectum. Results are usually available in about 2 days or sooner.

One in four pregnant people is a carrier of GBS, which means the bacteria are present in their bodily fluids but they show no signs of infection. Approximately 1 in 200 babies born to these people acquires a GBS infection, which can cause serious illnesses in the newborn, such as pneumonia, sepsis (infection in the blood), and meningitis. GBS infections in newborns can be almost entirely prevented by giving intravenous antibiotics to every laboring person who tests positive for Group B strep, after the membranes rupture or when they go into labor. The antibiotics, which reach the baby via the placenta, lower the risk of newborn infection to 1 in 2,000 to 4,000. The antibiotics also lower the pregnant person's risk of developing an active GBS infection, which may cause fever, uterine or urinary tract infection, and abdominal pain.

If a GBS carrier gives birth before receiving sufficient antibiotics, the baby is observed for symptoms of infection, tested for Group B strep, or both. The tests used vary among caregivers. Some rely on a blood culture only; others also culture the baby's urine and spinal fluid. Some caregivers treat all these babies with intravenous antibiotics and observe them closely for signs of infection for 2 to 3 days, until the tests are complete. Others watch the babies closely and treat only if the baby shows signs of infection before the test results come back. If Group B strep bacteria are present in the cultures, the intravenous (IV) antibiotic treatment continues for many days, during which the baby must remain in the hospital where the IV can be monitored and the baby can be watched for signs of infection.

Recently, a "risk-prediction model" has been developed that assesses the likelihood of an infection developing in the baby under these circumstances. The tool has made it possible to reliably identify those babies who are not at risk for developing a GBS infection. Those babies do not have to go through the antibiotic treatment. You might want to ask your caregiver about this new development. (See Resources, on page 190, for more information.)

The main disadvantage of GBS screening is that, if the pregnant person is a carrier, they not only must take intravenous antibiotics, but will probably also have labor induced if the membranes rupture without contractions. Several doses of antibiotics may be given during the waiting period. A common practice is to give a maximum of four doses and to plan induction if the pregnant person does not go into labor within 24 hours. Some caregivers are more patient than others under these circumstances, as are some pregnant people. Either choice—large amounts of antibiotics or induction—has disadvantages (see page 114).

Many people are relieved to learn that the antibiotics, although given intravenously, are administered only every 4 to 6 hours, depending on the antibiotic. Between doses, the IV line can be plugged and disconnected allowing the laboring person to move around. People planning an out-of-hospital birth do not have to switch to a hospital birth because of Group B strep, but they do have to visit their midwife every 4 to 6 hours for the antibiotics.

Most researchers agree there is need for better scientific research to determine the true value and potential harms of antibiotics in labor. Alternative treatments to prevent newborn infection, such as the use of probiotics, homeopathics, vaginal flushes, and others, have not been found effective, but also have not been adequately studied.

Ultrasonography

Ultrasonography is used for numerous purposes throughout pregnancy. In late pregnancy, it is used mostly to identify the baby's presentation when a breech or other difficult presentation is suspected, to estimate the baby's growth and weight, and to measure the volume of amniotic fluid. A decrease in fluid may indicate the placenta is no longer functioning very well; an increase may indicate a problem with the pregnant person's fluid regulation or the baby's kidneys. Unfortunately, the margin of error with these estimates can be considerable. For example, if somewhat dehydrated when a pregnant person has an ultrasound measurement of amniotic fluid volume, it is likely to be lower than if they were well hydrated. There's a lesson here: be sure they are well hydrated if having such a test.

Nonstress Test

This test assesses the baby's well-being by measuring heart rate changes that occur when the baby moves in the uterus. The nonstress test is recommended when the pregnant person notices the baby's movements slowing in frequency, when the caregiver feels the baby's growth may be less than expected, or when the pregnant person is overdue or has high blood pressure, diabetes, or another medical condition.

Using an external electronic fetal monitor (see page 108), the pregnant person presses a button when the baby moves. If the baby's heart rate speeds up, this is a good sign; the heart rate is said to be "reactive." If the rate stays the same or slows—if it is "nonreactive"— this may indicate the baby may be stressed, and further tests or corrective action may be necessary.

The nonstress test is not wholly accurate. When the test indicates the baby is doing well, it is usually correct. When it indicates the baby is not doing well, however, the results are often wrong. Combining a measurement of amniotic fluid volume with the nonstress test seems to give a more accurate picture of a baby's well-being.

ESSENTIAL OBSERVATIONS DURING LABOR

What constitutes basic care during labor when the laboring person is in good general health, has experienced a normal pregnancy, and the baby is in a favorable position within the uterus? By making certain simple observations regularly during the labor, the skilled caregiver or nurse can accurately assess whether both pregnant parent and baby are fine or whether closer observation or treatment is needed.

Basic care includes the following essential observations of the laboring person, labor progress, the amniotic fluid (the water in the bag of waters), the fetus, and the newborn.

The caregiver or nurse makes these observations of the **laboring person:**

- Behavior, activity, and emotional state during and between contractions and after the birth
- Basic body functions: eating, drinking, urination, bowel movements
- Contractions: frequency, intensity, and duration
- Tone of the uterus between contractions
- Location and nature of labor pain (abdomen, back, or both and whether the pain is continuous or intermittent)
- Rating the laboring person's pain (on a scale of 0 to 10). Most hospitals, by policy, assess every patient's level of pain and offer pain medication if the pain is increasing or distressing to the patient.
- Vaginal secretions
- Progress of labor (determined by the pattern of contractions, the patient's behavior, and occasional vaginal exams)
- Vital signs: temperature, pulse, and respiration
- Blood pressure
- Tone of the uterus after childbirth
- Amount of bleeding after childbirth

When the bag of waters breaks, the caregiver or nurse makes these observations of the **amniotic fluid:**

- Color: If the fluid is clear, the baby has probably not been stressed. A brown or green color indicates a fetal bowel movement (meconium), which means the baby has been stressed.
- Amount (leak or gush): Sudden loss of a large amount of fluid (a gush) increases the likelihood of pressure on the umbilical cord during contractions, which could cause stress to the baby.
- Odor: A foul smell indicates infection.
  The caregiver or nurse makes these observations of the **fetus:**
- Heartbeat, monitored by frequent listening with an ultrasound device (handheld or embedded in a belt around the abdomen) or a stethoscope
- Size (approximate weight)

The simple observations listed previously are made frequently by a caregiver or nurse who is with the laboring person nearly continuously. They give a very good idea of both the baby's and laboring person's condition. As long as they indicate normal conditions, these observations are all that is truly needed. If they indicate problems with the laboring person, the labor, or the baby, then additional interventions (described in the next pages) are used to correct the problems.

Immediately after birth, the caregiver or nurse makes these observations of the **newborn**. They are a quick assessment of the newborn's well-being:

- Baby's temperature, respiration, and pulse
- Baby's general behavior and state of alertness
- Baby's physical appearance
- Apgar score at 1, 5, and, perhaps, 10 minutes after birth

APGAR SCORE (ASSESSED AT 1, 5, AND, SOMETIMES, 10 MINUTES)

SIGN	0 points	1 point	2 points
Heart rate	Absent	below 100 per minute	more than 100 per minute
Breathing	Absent	slow, irregular	good, crying
Muscle tone	Limp	arms and legs close to body	active, moving
Reflex irritability	no response to mild pinch	Grimace	struggle, cough, or sneeze
Color	blue-gray	body usual skin color; fingers and toes blue	all pink or ruddy

A score of 7 to 10 at 1 and 5 minutes of age is considered good health. Below 7 indicates the baby needs attention, such as suctioning their mouth and nose; giving oxygen or other aid to breathing; rubbing and stroking the baby's skin; or having the parents speak or sing to the baby. Lower scores indicate the need for more skilled medical care.

CONDITIONS INFLUENCING THE USE OF INTERVENTION DURING LABOR

Beyond the essential observations already discussed, other tests, procedures, and medications are used if potential problems are discovered. They include the use of highly specialized equipment, a variety of drugs, and surgery. How and when they are used depends on a number of considerations:

- Medical condition of the pregnant parent: As already noted, there is less need for intervention when the pregnant parent experiences a healthy pregnancy, labor is progressing well, and all vital signs are normal.
- Apparent well-being of the fetus: If the fetus is fully developed and mature, of normal size, and apparently unstressed, most interventions are not needed.
- Training and philosophy of the caregiver: Some caregivers routinely use more interventions than others, preferring to prevent problems before they arise. Although this results in unnecessary treatment, these caregivers feel that overtreatment is harmless and that without it, they might miss problems. Better safe than sorry, they believe. Oth-

er caregivers are comfortable watching the laboring person, baby, and labor progress and using interventions only if a problem arises; they believe unnecessary treatment can cause problems. The scientific literature supports the latter approach.

- Usual practices or policies of the institution and nursing staff: These practices or policies are determined by current standards of care, nurses' training, the size and competence of the staff, customs in the hospital, legal concerns, financial considerations, and other factors. There is much variation in usual practices among hospitals—even in the same geographical area. In one hospital, for example, laboring people may be encouraged to be out of bed and moving about or using the bath in labor. In another hospital nearby, they may be discouraged from doing these same things. Rates of labor induction, epidural analgesia, and cesarean delivery also vary widely among hospitals.
- Preferences of the pregnant person: Within each institution and within each caregiver's practice, there is room for choice. Make sure the caregiver knows the pregnant person's preferences; help ensure their preferences are considered in all decisions made.

COMMON OBSTETRIC INTERVENTIONS

Following are descriptions of many common obstetric procedures and their purposes, disadvantages, and possible alternatives. These are usually unnecessary when labor is normal, but may become necessary if problems arise. Chapter 7 discusses the circumstances under which these procedures are necessary for medical reasons.

As the birth partner, you may be the liaison between the laboring person and the hospital staff. A doula can advise you in this role. It is important for you to be familiar with common obstetric interventions so you can inform the staff about the laboring person's preferences, help them make decisions about optional procedures, and help handle any additional discomfort—emotional or physical—arising from the interventions. It is also important that you both understand any circumstances that require interventions for safety.

Intravenous (IV) Fluids

An intravenous (IV) drip is a plastic bag that includes water and electrolytes, dextrose, or medication. The liquid runs from a plastic bag to a needle. A tube extends from the bag and is inserted into a vein in the laboring person's hand or arm. The liquid drips into the vein.

REASONS FOR GIVING IV FLUIDS DURING SOME LABORS

IV fluids provide liquids, calories, and/or medications without having to swallow them; with an epidural, to increase blood volume to help protect against a drop in blood pressure; or to keep a vein open, in case medications are required quickly later in labor.

Some caregivers recognize that routine IV fluids are problematic and instead encourage laboring people to drink enough fluids to satisfy their thirst. IV fluids are reserved for times when they are "medically indicated"—that is, when necessary or desirable because of the medical condition of the laboring person or baby, such as when:

- Labor is very long.
- The person has severe vomiting and dehydration.
- They will receive epidural, spinal, or general anesthesia (see pages 139–142).

- They need IV medications: e.g., to stop preterm labor, induce or speed labor, control blood pressure, reduce pain, or other reasons.
- They have a condition that might require immediate medical action.

DISADVANTAGES OF GIVING IV FLUIDS

Some caregivers give IV fluids to all laboring patients instead of allowing them to eat and drink to keep the stomach empty. This practice is left over from when most people gave birth while unconscious under general anesthesia. They might vomit and breathe in any stomach contents. General anesthesia is now rarely used and, when it is, safer techniques protect against this complication. Nevertheless, some doctors continue to withhold food and drink. Large amounts of IV fluids cause fluid retention in the laboring person, especially in the legs and breasts. It may take days for this to disappear, and the increase in breast engorgement makes breastfeeding more difficult during the first week. In addition:

- An IV line is inconvenient and somewhat stressful for the laboring person, who must make sure it is out of the way when rolling over or getting out of bed.
- IV lines sometimes "infiltrate"—that is, poke through the vein. The fluids then go directly into the laboring person's tissue, causing pain and swelling. If the fluids contain medications, they do no good, as they do not get into the bloodstream.
  Here are some alternatives to IV fluids that you can discuss with the caregiver:
- After every contraction or two, offer the laboring person fluids, such as water, juice, coconut water, sports beverages, or frozen juice bars There is no need to urge them to drink large amounts. The person's thirst is usually a good guide. The nurse also watches the person's intake and can detect possible dehydration.

If the caregiver wants the option to give IV medications quickly, a heparin lock or saline flush may be used. A thin flexible tube is placed in the vein, but not connected to an IV line. This allows the laboring person to move freely, while enabling a quick connection to IV fluids, if needed.

Electronic Fetal Monitoring (EFM)

There are three methods of electronic fetal monitoring (EFM): external, internal, and portable external.

With external monitoring, two devices are placed on the person's abdomen. One, an ultrasound device that detects the fetal heartbeat, is placed low on the abdomen where the heartbeat can be best detected. The second, a tocodynamometer (usually called "toco" for short) that detects contractions, is placed higher on the abdomen, They are held in place, either by stretchy belts around abdomen, or by adhesive patches that stick the devices to the abdomen. The patches are less widely used, but more comfortable, as they are not tightly wrapped around the abdomen. With internal fetal monitoring, a thin spiral wire electrode is attached to the skin of the baby's scalp to detect the fetal heart rate electronically. A fluid-filled tube, called an intrauterine pressure catheter, may also be placed within the laboring person's uterus to measure the intensity of the contractions.

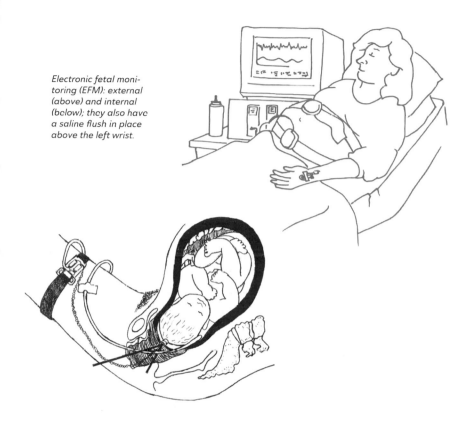

Electronic fetal monitoring (EFM): external (above) and internal (below); they also have a saline flush in place above the left wrist.

The information about contractions and the baby's heart rate response to them is transmitted either by wires to a bedside display or wirelessly to a screen at the nurses' station. The readings can also be printed out continuously.

With *portable electronic fetal monitoring* (telemetry), the laboring person may wear a radio transmitter around their neck, which connects by short wires to the sensors in the belts (instead of wires connected to the bedside console). Or, they may use a newer wireless version. In these, radio transmitters are located within each sensor, and the sensors are waterproof, so the laboring person can be monitored in the water. Either type allows the laboring person to move about freely (within about 200 feet, or 61 meters, of the nurses' station) while information is radioed back to a central monitor and the monitor in the labor room. External monitoring is easier to apply, less invasive, and much more widely used than internal monitoring, but the latter is more accurate and reserved for times when external monitoring is not tracking the fetal heartbeat or the contractions accurately enough (as with a laboring person who is also obese, contractions of questionable intensity, and other situations).

PURPOSES OF EFM DURING LABOR

EFM detects, displays, and records the baby's heart rate response to contractions. A permanent record of the length, frequency, and (with internal monitoring) intensity of the contractions, along with the fetal heart rate, is produced.

EFM is **medically indicated** during labor when:

- Synthetic oxytocin is used to induce or speed up labor (see page 115). The length and frequency of the contractions can be assessed with the external tocodynamometer. If the caregiver needs an accurate measurement of the intensity of the contractions, the intrauterine pressure catheter is used.
- A nurse or a midwife cannot be with the laboring person continuously or frequently.
- There are doubts during labor about the fetus's well-being (because of prematurity, small size, meconium-stained amniotic fluid, or possible lack of oxygen).
- The laboring person is considered to be at high risk for complications.

Disadvantages of EFM are:

- The laboring person's movements are restricted, although they can change position in bed and sometimes even stand by the bed or sit in a chair. Portable monitoring allows for more movement, including walking around, and wireless monitoring is possible while in a bath or shower. Internal monitoring is less restrictive but more invasive than external monitoring.
- Sometimes, more attention is paid to the machine than the laboring person. As the birth partner, do not allow yourself to fall into this trap. The laboring person needs your attention, not the machine.
- Interpretation of the monitor printouts (tracings) is extremely complex, and experts even disagree about what different heart rate patterns really mean and when intervention is necessary.
- Internal monitoring requires breaking both the bag of waters and the skin of the fetal scalp. These procedures slightly increase the risk of infection to the laboring person and baby, especially if the laboring person has an infection or sore in the vagina. Also, breaking the bag of waters may cause additional stress to the fetus by removing the cushion of fluid that protects the head and cord.
- EFM measures only the fetal pulse, but it cannot detect whether the fetus is experiencing a shortage of oxygen. When cesareans are done solely because of EFM tracings, the babies often show no signs of having been oxygen deprived. For this reason, attempts to confirm the findings of EFM are sometimes used (see "Fetal Scalp Stimulation Test," page 111).

Alternatives to consider: Before labor, you and the pregnant person can discuss the following alternatives to EFM and state your preferences in your birth plan.

- Have a nurse or midwife listen frequently to fetal heart tones with an ultrasound stethoscope or a fetal stethoscope, for 1 to 2 minutes at a time during and after a contraction. Many studies have compared this method of monitoring with continuous EFM, and all have found that listening to heart tones intermittently results in equally healthy babies and fewer cesareans. This method, called auscultation, requires the nurse or midwife to be trained and experienced and be available for about 5 minutes out of every 15 during active labor and continuously during the birthing stage. Auscultation is the method used in home or out-of-hospital birth centers.

- Use external EFM intermittently for 10 to 15 minutes each hour, removing it the rest of the time. This enables the laboring person to move around when not being monitored. Some caregivers are comfortable doing this in early labor, but prefer continuous monitoring in active labor and beyond.
- Use a portable (telemetry) EFM unit (see page 108). Find out whether the hospital has portable telemetry units available.
- Use a handheld waterproof ultrasound stethoscope or the waterproof telemetry units for listening to the baby when the laboring person is in the bath. These are not available in all hospitals. Ask the caregiver about them.

Fetal Scalp Stimulation Test

The caregiver performs this simple test by pressing or scratching the baby's scalp during a vaginal exam. If the baby is in good condition, the heart rate will speed up with such stimulation. If the baby is distressed (that is, short of oxygen), the heart rate will not speed up. The results of this test have been found to correlate well with the actual condition of the fetus.

This test is performed to check whether the baby is still tolerating labor even though the EFM tracings or audible heart sounds raise concerns. The test is medically indicated at any time fetal heart tones are unclear (the medical terms for this are "nonreassuring" or "indeterminate," meaning there is concern about the baby's well-being) and certainly before a cesarean is performed for fetal intolerance of labor (which is considered to be diagnostic of oxygen deprivation). This simple test can be performed any number of times during labor.

Alternatives to consider Instead of performing the fetal scalp stimulation test, you can simply rely on EFM alone or on frequent listening to the fetal heart rate, which may result in overcalling fetal intolerance of labor.

You and the laboring person can ask for the fetal scalp stimulation test whenever fetal distress is suspected. Discuss it with the caregiver in advance and state your preference for it in the birth plan.

Artificial Rupture of the Membranes (AROM)

To rupture the membranes, or break the bag of waters, the caregiver inserts a thin instrument (amnihook) into the vagina and through the cervix and makes a hole in the sac holding the amniotic fluid, which then comes streaming out. The procedure is no more painful than a vaginal exam. Sometimes, following AROM, the laboring person's contractions suddenly increase in intensity; this is usually the goal of the procedure.

In the past, laboring people were warned against taking baths after their membranes were ruptured, but scientific trials have found that bathing in a clean tub after AROM does not increase the chance of infection in either the laboring person or the baby.

AROM is done:

- To speed labor. If timed correctly and the baby is well positioned, AROM shortens labor by an average of 40 minutes. If the baby is malpositioned, however, the procedure may actually lengthen labor. Rupturing the membranes removes the cushion of fluid around the baby's head, and may cause the malpositioned head to wedge more firmly into the pelvis, which lessens the chances that the baby's position will improve. It cannot always be predicted which labors will be shortened by AROM and which will not. The gamble may be worth taking when labor progress is poor because other interventions to speed labor are more complex and potentially risky.
- To induce labor with other methods, such as prostaglandins or oxytocin (see pages 114–115). AROM alone is not likely to induce labor unless the cervix is very soft and thin.
- To check the amniotic fluid for a fetal bowel movement (meconium, which can signal fetal stress), for infection, for bleeding, or for other signs of problems
- To apply the electrode and catheter for internal EFM (see page 108)
- When is AROM medically indicated? This question is controversial. The frequency with which caregivers use AROM, especially in early labor, varies widely. Some believe it is innocuous and use it for most of their patients in labor. Others believe its advantages rarely outweigh its disadvantages; they reserve it for situations in which they feel they must intervene. Otherwise, they prefer to leave the membranes intact.

Disadvantages of AROM are:

- It may not start or speed labor.
- Chances of infection for the laboring person or baby increase with time after the bag of waters is broken and with the number of vaginal exams performed.
- Removing the protective cushion of fluid from around the baby's head may increase pressure on the head during contractions and cause indeterminate or nonreassuring fetal heart rate changes.
- If the baby's head is malpositioned, removing the thin fluid layer surrounding the head may take away any wiggle room, thereby decreasing the chance of the head repositioning.
- AROM increases the risk that the umbilical cord will be compressed during contractions. This compression could cause fetal heart rate changes that indicate a shortage of oxygen for the baby.
- If the baby's head (or buttocks, if the baby is breech) is high when AROM is done, the danger of a prolapsed cord (see page 131) increases.

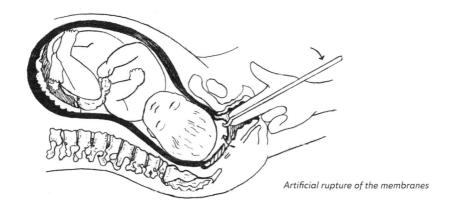

Artificial rupture of the membranes

Alternatives to consider:

- The caregiver can refrain from breaking the bag of waters to speed labor and suggest that the laboring person try self-help methods to stimulate contractions (see pages 90–96).
- Or, they can use other methods to check fetal well-being (see "Electronic Fetal Monitoring," page 108 and "Fetal Scalp Stimulation Test," page 111) or to induce labor.

Amnioinfusion

In this painless procedure, saline solution (salty water) is sent into the uterus via a plastic tube, the same kind used with an intrauterine pressure catheter to assess the intensity of contractions. Amnioinfusion is done after the bag of waters has broken to replace the fluid lost if the baby's umbilical cord is being compressed during contractions.

The added fluid helps cushion the cord and may protect against fetal distress. The procedure is also helpful if the baby has passed meconium in the uterus. The fluid dilutes the meconium to protect against problems that would occur if the baby were to inhale thick meconium during birth. Although the injected fluid gradually runs out of the uterus, the procedure can be repeated as necessary to maintain sufficient volume. This simple technique, which is extremely low cost, sometimes makes it possible to safely avoid a cesarean for fetal intolerance of labor.

Disadvantages of amnioinfusion are:
- It is invasive and can increase the chance of uterine infection.
- The laboring person must remain flat in bed during and after the procedure or the fluid will run out quickly.

Alternatives to consider:
- The caregiver can go straight to a cesarean when fetal distress warrants quick delivery.

Induction or Augmentation of Labor

Sometimes, labor is induced (started artificially) and at other times, a labor that has slowed is augmented (speeded up). There are several ways labor can be induced or augmented:

1. Self-help methods (see pages 54–64)

2. "Stripping" the membranes to begin labor induction. The caregiver inserts a finger in the vagina through the cervix and circles the finger around inside to separate the membranes from the lower segment of the uterus. This is usually uncomfortable or painful for the pregnant person—it feels like a vigorous vaginal exam—and sometimes results in inadvertent rupture of the membranes. Stripping the membranes usually does not actually start labor, but it may hasten ripening and thinning of the cervix to make it more ready for dilation (see "Labor Progresses in Six Ways," page 24). The procedure cannot be done if the cervix is hard to reach because it is very posterior (pointing toward the pregnant person's back) instead of anterior (in the center of the vagina) or if it is tightly closed.

3. Artificial rupture of the membranes (AROM, see page 111). This sometimes speeds or augments labor when timed correctly.

4. Prostaglandin gels, suppositories, or tablets. Prostaglandins are hormone-like substances produced by the body. They can also be manufactured. Like the prostaglandins a pregnant person produces, synthetic prostaglandins promote the softening, thinning, and, sometimes, dilation of the cervix. They are used when labor must be induced before the cervix has naturally softened or thinned. Prostaglandins come in these forms:

   - A water-soluble gel containing prostaglandin (dinoprostone or Prepidil), applied to the inside or the outside of the cervix through a syringe. This may be repeated after 6 hours or so.

   - A tampon-like device containing prostaglandin (Cervidil), placed in the vagina behind the cervix, where it gradually releases prostaglandin over about 12 hours

   - A tiny tablet containing another synthetic prostaglandin, misoprostol (Cytotec), either placed in the vagina behind the cervix or given by mouth. Tablets are given by mouth when a pregnant person's membranes have ruptured because placing anything in the vagina increases the risk of infection. A second tablet may be administered after 4 to 6 hours. Cytotec should be given in low doses (25 micrograms vaginally or 50 micrograms orally) and usually acts gradually, as Prepidil and Cervidil do. Higher doses can cause sudden, very intense, contractions and fetal distress. This is less likely to happen with dinoprostone or Prepidil.

     These agents are only used in the hospital and require careful observation of the pregnant person and fetus for unwanted side effects. Dosages and treatment schedules vary depending on the caregiver's preferences, the pregnant person's preferences, and the state of the cervix. Lower doses are generally safer but act more slowly.

5. Intravenous administration of a synthetic form of the hormone oxytocin (also called Pitocin) can start or speed up labor. Pitocin is mixed with intravenous fluids in a continuous drip. By regulating the dose, the caregiver can usually control the intensity and frequency of the contractions quite well. Electronic fetal monitoring is required, along with a nurse's close observation, to detect and correct excessively strong or long contractions. Attempts to start labor with Pitocin often fail when the cervix is firm and thick. If prostaglandin is used before Pitocin, this problem is often avoided.

If an induction is done for medical reasons and fails, cesarean delivery is the only remaining option. If an induction is done without a medical reason (that is, for convenience) and fails, the pregnant person may be sent home to await spontaneous labor, but this rarely happens today. Usually, the baby is delivered by cesarean.

Induction or augmentation of labor is **medically indicated** when:

- Pregnancy is prolonged. Caregivers disagree about when pregnancy has gone on too long. Some offer induction at 39, 40, or 41 weeks, but there is scientific evidence that, statistically, if there is no medical problem, the risks to the baby of inducing before 42 weeks exceed the risks of waiting. However, waiting beyond 42 or 43 weeks increases the risk of stillbirth. In 2016, the American College of Obstetricians and Gynecologists recommended that, without a medical reason, induction of labor should be postponed until 42 weeks of pregnancy.
- Medical problems are such that continuing the pregnancy might harm the pregnant person or the baby (for example, when the pregnant person has high blood pressure or diabetes).
- The baby is not thriving in the uterus.
- The bag of waters has been broken for a long time and labor has not started spontaneously or the pregnant person has tested positive for Group B strep (see page103).
- The pregnant person who has frequent herpes outbreaks is free of herpes sore in the genital area. Being induced is a way to avoid a cesarean (which is done if a pregnant person has a herpes sore in or near the vagina when going into labor; see page 127).
- The pregnant person is having a prolonged prelabor and the cervix is firm, in which case the use of prostaglandins may be appropriate (see "Prelabor," page 29 and "The Slow-to-Start Labor," page 92).
- Contractions in the active phase slow and decrease in intensity, causing a delay in progress. In this case, augmentation with intravenous Pitocin may be appropriate.

Disadvantages of induction for medical reasons include:

- Medical induction usually includes more interventions for safety than does spontaneous onset of labor; such interventions include continuous electronic fetal monitoring, IV fluids, and others.
- Because the pregnant person is hospitalized before the first contraction—possibly hours before—they can become tired and hungry, perhaps discouraged, and even begin to perceive that their labor is very long and something is wrong.

Sometimes, labor is induced out of fear that the baby is becoming too big. The reasoning is, inducing labor before the baby grows too much will make the birth easier and prevent complications and, possibly, a cesarean. Although this seems to make sense, studies have shown that:

- It is not possible to assess an unborn baby's size accurately. Estimates are often wrong by 10 percent or more, even when ultrasound is used.
- When babies are thought to be large, cesareans are more likely if labor is induced than if labor begins spontaneously, and induction, in these cases, produces no improvements in the babies' health and well-being.
- Although the odds of a difficult labor increase when the baby's weight exceeds 8½ pounds (3.9 kilograms), inducing labor does not prevent a difficult labor or a cesarean birth.
- Most cases of shoulder dystocia (in which a baby becomes stuck after the head is out) happen in average-size babies; this problem cannot be predicted. When this serious complication occurs, doctors and midwives use well-practiced techniques to resolve it.

Nonmedical reasons for induction: While it is difficult to quantify exactly, many inductions are elective; that is, not for medical safety but for reasons such as:

- Convenience—for the pregnant person, caregiver, or both. An elective induction may be scheduled to occur when the caregiver is on call or when the pregnant person has household help.
- Routine procedure, whenever a pregnant person reaches week 39 or 40. Many caregivers see no reason not to induce labor at this point, and they are not concerned about the possibility of prematurity or the increased likelihood of a cesarean (see disadvantages, following).
- The pregnant person's discomfort. Swelling, backache, itching, or fatigue makes some women want to end their pregnancies as soon as safety allows.
- Avoiding the stress of traveling to the hospital in labor, especially if the pregnant person lives far from the hospital or has had a previous rapid labor.

It can be very appealing to be able to plan when the baby will be born. As the birth partner, you might appreciate knowing the date and being able to plan your schedule accordingly. However, inductions are more successful if done when the cervix has already ripened (softened and thinned) considerably.

Disadvantages of elective induction: Because induction is not an innocuous procedure, you and the pregnant person should carefully consider the benefits and risks of an elective induction before ceciding. There are many potential disadvantages:

1. Inductions sometimes proceed very slowly, especially if the pregnant person's cervix has not undergone some of the dilation changes (see "Labor Progresses in Six Ways," page 24). A day or more may pass before the baby is born, and, in some cases, the induction procedures are carried out during the day and stopped at night

to allow the pregnant person to eat and get some rest. The reason for allowing plenty of time for the process is to try to avoid a cesarean; however, a slow induction can be exhausting and demoralizing for both the pregnant person and birth partner. (If the bag of waters has broken, the caregiver usually intervenes with a cesarean earlier.) Some caregivers are reluctant to put the pregnant person through a long induction or to wait several days for the birth, and so they decide on a cesarean after 12 hours or so, although labor may not have even begun in this much time. You may wonder if the induction for no medical reason is worth these risks.

2. The timing of an elective induction may not be best for the baby, who might benefit from another few days or weeks in the uterus. Most babies continue to mature and develop greater strength and other capabilities until labor begins spontaneously. Normally, the baby, when mature enough, starts the labor process, by secreting the hormones that initiate labor. If the pregnant person's due date is uncertain and labor is induced, the baby might be premature. In fact, elective induction has been identified as one large and preventable contributor to the high rate of prematurity (10 percent) in the United States.

3. Prostaglandins used to ripen the cervix sometimes cause nausea and rapid changes in the pregnant person's blood pressure.

4. The chances of a cesarean are greater in a first-time pregnant person who has an elective induction compared to a first-time pregnant person whose labor begins spontaneously.

5. Sometimes, even though the induction date is planned, the hospital is too busy or lacking an available bed when the day comes. The pregnant person may be told not to come in or may even be turned away on arrival. They may be asked to call the hospital every few hours until a bed becomes available. This can be frustrating and worrisome, especially if they have not been warned that this could happen or if they think the induction was suggested for medical reasons.

6. Induced labors may cause contractions that are too long or too strong for the baby (or the pregnant person) to tolerate. Sometimes, the staff, in the desire for a fast labor, may begin with contractions that are much stronger than natural contractions and that could harm the baby. To detect such a problem, the pregnant person must have continuous electronic fetal monitoring (see page 108). To protect against this happening, you can ask the staff to start and increase the contractions gradually—more like a natural labor.

If the laboring person's contractions are too strong for the baby to tolerate well, the nurse takes measures to stop them. If the laboring person is receiving intravenous Pitocin, the nurse can turn it off or turn it down; the contractions, usually, quickly subside. If the laboring person has had prostaglandin placed in the vagina, the nurse either removes the insert (Cervidil) or washes out the gel (Prepidil) or the tablet (Cytotec). If the pregnant person has swallowed a Cytotec tablet, another drug, such as Terbutaline, may be given to slow the contractions.

7. Use of pain medications early in the dilation process is more likely with induction, for several reasons:

- The laboring person may be restricted from using comfort measures, such as changing positions, walking, and massage, by the intravenous line and the electronic fetal monitor's belts and cords.
- Fatigue and discouragement over a slow onset of labor may lower the laboring person's motivation to deal with the contractions. They also may feel hungry, as they may not be allowed to eat before or while the Pitocin is being given. (A request to eat lightly is a good item for the birth plan, though some hospitals routinely deny food in labor.)
- As said earlier, with induced labor, Pitocin may be given in high enough doses to cause stronger and more frequent contractions than those that usually occur in noninduced labors. Contractions in early labor (before 4 or 5 centimeters) may be more difficult to handle than if labor began spontaneously.
- If the pregnant person is hospitalized before contractions start, the labor seems much longer and slower than if labor begins at home where they can keep busy with normal activities. They might become concerned that labor is going too slowly and lose confidence in the ability to handle it.

Although medically indicated induction has some of the same disadvantages, knowing there is good reason for the induction makes these disadvantages more acceptable.

Alternatives to consider: If there is *no medical reason* for induction, you and the pregnant person can:

- Wait for spontaneous labor. If the pregnant person asks about postponing an elective induction, the caregiver may be willing to wait for labor to start on its own, at least until they are 1 to 2 weeks past the due date—as long as there is careful surveillance of the pregnant person's and baby's well-being.
- Try the nonmedical methods for stimulating labor contractions described on pages 90–96, "When Labor Must Start"

Episiotomy

An episiotomy is a surgical cut, made with scissors, from the vagina toward the anus shortly before delivery. Anesthesia may be given before the procedure, but, even if done without anesthesia, the birthing person is hardly aware of it. Rather than feeling pain, there maybe relief from the stretching and burning sensation when the episiotomy is performed. Local anesthesia is given after the birth to relieve pain that occurs when the episiotomy is stitched. The incision usually heals within 1 to 2 weeks, although pain at the site may linger, during physical exertion and intercourse, for weeks or, rarely, months. If there is still pain after a few weeks, consult the caregiver.

Once routine, episiotomies are rarely performed by midwives; physicians also do far fewer now than in the early and mid-1990s. The main reason for doing an episiotomy was to avoid a tear in the perineum (the area between the vagina and the anus) or in the front of the vagina. Episiotomies became less common when scientific evidence showed that this rationale was unsupportable (see disadvantages, below).

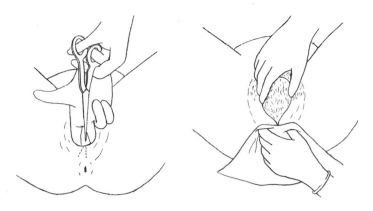

Episiotomy. The midline incision is most common in the United States.

Purposes of episiotomy are:

- To speed delivery by 5 to 10 minutes, if the baby appears severely compromised
- To reduce pressure on the baby's head, if the baby is premature or has other problems
- To enlarge a very tight vaginal opening, when necessary, to allow delivery. It is very rare that the vagina will not stretch adequately.
- To allow easier placement of forceps

Disadvantages of episiotomy: An episiotomy will *definitely* damage the birthing person's perineum—they will have a cut, stitches, a healing period, and some discomfort or pain. If no episiotomy is done, however, there is about a 30 to 60 percent chance that the birthing person's perineum will have a tear. Research indicates that spontaneous tears are almost always smaller, require fewer stitches, and are quicker to heal than the average episiotomy.

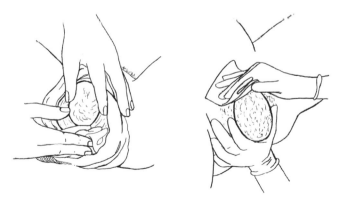

Normal delivery without episiotomy, with the birthing person on their side. Left: The caregiver uses warm compresses to promote relaxation and circulation and gently supports the perineum. Right: With the birthing person rolled toward their side, the caregiver provides slight counterpressure as the baby's head emerges.

In addition, episiotomies sometimes *extend*—that is, after the cut is made, the pressure of the baby's head can enlarge the incision. This happens in approximately 1 person in 20. Spontaneous tears are rarely (fewer than 1 in 100) as large as extended episiotomies. In other words, the chance of a serious tear is greater *with* an episiotomy than without.

Alternatives to consider: The caregiver can simply forego an episiotomy, even if it appears that the birthing person may tear. They may incur no injury, one or several small tears, or, rarely, a tear as large as an average episiotomy (rarely larger).

The caregiver can protect the perineum from tearing seriously—for example, by placing warm compresses on the perineum, controlling the birth of the head and shoulders, suggesting positions that facilitate the baby's descent, and allowing spontaneous rather than directed bearing down (see "The Crowning and Birth Phase," page 48, and "Spontaneous Bearing Down," page 65).

You and the birthing person can improve the chance of an intact perineum after birth by doing prenatal perineal massage (see page 80).

Whether or not a birthing person ends up with a perineal tear or an episiotomy, exercising the pelvic floor muscles after birth seems to be very important to the recovery of pelvic floor tone; see page 10 for a discussion of the Kegel exercises.

Vacuum Extraction

Vacuum extraction is sometimes used during the birthing (second) stage of labor, only after the birthing person has pushed for a long time without progress. A silicone suction cup (about 3 inches, or 7.5 cm, in diameter) is placed in the vagina on the baby's head. The suction cup is connected to a handle and a pump that creates a safe level of suction. The caregiver pulls on the device attached to the baby's head while the uterus contracts and the birthing person pushes. Once the baby's head is out, the suction cup is removed and the birthing person pushes the baby out. An important safety measure is that the suction cup comes off if the caregiver pulls too hard, thus protecting the baby's head. If the vacuum doesn't succeed, a cesarean becomes necessary.

Vacuum extraction is done to assist or hasten delivery after the baby's head is in the birth canal. This procedure is **medically indicated** if:

- The birthing (second) stage of labor is prolonged because fatigue or anesthesia has made it difficult for the birthing person to push effectively.
- The birthing stage is prolonged because the baby's head is angled or very large so it doesn't fit through the pelvis, and the birthing person's efforts need assistance.
- There is last-minute fetal distress.

Compared with forceps (see following), vacuum extraction less often requires an episiotomy, may cause less damage to the birthing person's vagina, and appears to be about equally safe for the baby.

Disadvantages of vacuum extraction are:
- Vacuum extraction frequently causes a fluid-filled lump and a bruise or abrasion on the baby's head where the suction cup was. It may take days or weeks for the lump to disappear.

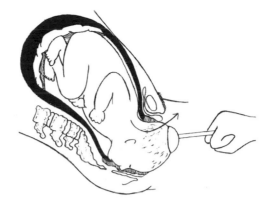

Vacuum extraction. After applying a suction cup to the baby's scalp, the caregiver pulls as the birthing person pushes and the uterus contracts.

- Serious injury to the baby's head is possible, though very unlikely when the vacuum extractor is used according to safety guidelines set by the Food and Drug Administration (FDA) and the obstetric profession.
- If the suction cup pops off during use, both the birth partner and the birthing person may be alarmed. Remember, it pops off to protect the baby from excessive strain.

Alternatives to consider:
- The birthing person can bear down (push) in different positions, such as squatting or standing (see "Positions and Movements for Labor and Birth," pages 67–76).
- Forceps can be used for delivery (see "Forceps Delivery," following).
- A cesarean delivery can be performed (see chapter 9).

Forceps Delivery

Forceps are used late in the birthing stage to deliver the baby more quickly. Two steel instruments, like spoons or salad tongs, are placed, one at a time, within the vagina on either side of the baby's head. They are then locked together into position so the forceps cannot squeeze the baby's head, no matter how hard the doctor grips the handles. This protects the baby's head from undue pressure. The doctor pulls during contractions while the birthing person pushes. Sometimes, forceps are used to rotate the baby's head.

A forceps delivery is **medically indicated** when birth is delayed because the birthing person is not able to push effectively; there is a decrease in uterine contractions; or the baby is large or poorly positioned.

Forceps are also **medically indicated** if the baby is distressed when low in the birth canal. If the baby is too high in the birth canal for the safe use of forceps, a cesarean delivery (see chapter 9) is a safer choice than forceps.

If a forceps delivery appears difficult, the attempt is abandoned, and a cesarean is performed.

Disadvantages of forceps delivery are:
- A forceps delivery usually requires an episiotomy and anesthesia.
- Forceps may bruise the baby's face or the side of the head.

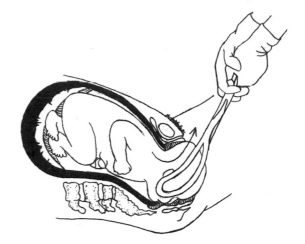

Forceps are placed in the birthing person's vagina around the baby's head. The doctor pulls while the mother pushes and the uterus contracts.

- Though rare, forceps may injure the baby's head or neck, especially if used with excessive force and contrary to the professional guidelines for the safe use of forceps.
- Forceps may injure the birthing person's vagina.

Alternatives to consider:

- If able to change positions, the birthing person can use directed pushing in positions that enlarge the pelvis, such as squatting with or without support, the dangle, rocking forward and back on hands and knees, or lying flat on their back and pulling the knees up toward the shoulders (see "Positions and Movements for Labor and Birth," pages 67–76 and "Directed Pushing," page 65).
- The caregiver can monitor the baby and birthing person; if both are doing well, they can give the labor more time.
- The caregiver can use vacuum extraction (see page 120). The choice between forceps and vacuum extraction is best made by the doctor, according to their training and expertise.
- The caregiver can attempt a forceps delivery once or twice, but, if it appears the baby is not moving, the caregiver removes the forceps and prepare for a cesarean.
- The doctor can perform a cesarean delivery. This is the only alternative if vacuum extraction does not work and a forceps delivery is not appropriate.

In summary, the purpose of medical interventions is to improve birth outcomes for the birthing person and baby. Most interventions carry some risks or disadvantages along with benefits. Therefore, they should be used only when needed.

Except in emergency circumstances, there is usually more than one way to accomplish the intended purpose of any proposed intervention. For this reason, you and the birthing person will want to be prepared to make informed choices about which options might be used and when

CHAPTER 7

Complications in Late Pregnancy, Labor, or Afterward

THIS CHAPTER DISCUSSES A NUMBER OF COMPLICATIONS that may arise before, during, or after labor, how they are treated, and how you can help the laboring person if they occur. More serious than the difficulties discussed in chapter 5, these complications require hospitalization and medical assistance for a good outcome. They fall into four major categories: problems with the laboring person; problems with the labor; problems with the fetus; and problems with the newborn.

Sometimes, the pregnant person or couples cannot have all their other priorities met because their most important priority—a healthy birthing person and healthy baby after the birth—requires accepting some interventions they hadn't previously wanted.

If the situation is serious and a quick decision must be made, the single most important question to ask the caregiver is: Will this (procedure, medicine, or treatment) improve our chances for a healthy birthing person and baby after the birth?

If the answer is yes, the answer is clear, and other priorities take a back seat. If no, you have time to consider options, using the Key Questions for Informed Decision-Making (page 101).

As the birth partner, you can help in the following ways:

- Learn what is happening, why it is a problem, how serious it is, and the rationale for and the expected results of any corrective action to be taken. Ask the caregiver the key questions (page 101), adding the most important question just noted. Help the pregnant person understand the answers.
- Remain assertive and cooperative with the caregiver. Inform the staff of the laboring person's wishes and learn any alternative ways of handling the problem. Use the birth plan (see page 11) as your guide.
- Recognize the need to accept the caregiver's judgment without discussion if there is a true emergency—when time is of the utmost importance.
- Help the pregnant person adjust to the need for a change in management. If the birth plan reflects the understanding that complications sometimes arise unexpectedly, they will realize a departure from some previous preferences is warranted to ensure a good

outcome for both the baby and themselves. A doula can help you both ask the right questions, adjust to the change in management, and maintain perspective.

- Remain with the laboring person throughout. When things go wrong, they need your help and support more than ever.
- Afterwards, allow them time to recover emotionally. You will also need time to recover.

COMPLICATIONS FOR THE PREGNANT PERSON

This section includes brief explanations of complications and why they are problematic; how the pregnant person may react; and how you can help. use the key questions to learn information about your care provider's management, and the information below about how to support the person in labor.

Premature (Preterm) Labor

Labor is premature if it begins before 37 weeks of pregnancy (see "Signs of Labor," page 21, for an explanation of signs of premature labor). If a pregnant person suspects they are having premature labor, call their caregiver for a diagnosis and advice. Early treatment sometimes stops premature labor. Babies born prematurely are at greater risk for a number of medical problems, such as breathing difficulties, jaundice, infection, difficulty maintaining body temperature, and feeding problems.

HOW THE PREGNANT PERSON MAY REACT

Both you and the pregnant person will be eager to do everything possible to help the baby get a healthy start in life. The pregnant person may feel guilt and self-blame that, in some way, they caused the contractions or if reduced activity or bed rest prevents them from doing their share of running the household. They may feel concerned about adding pressure on you. They may worry how a lengthy period of bed rest will affect their strength and fitness (if so, the caregivers may be able to recommend a physical therapist who can visit your home and teach some safe in-bed exercises). The pregnant person may become very bored lying around all the time.

HOW YOU CAN HELP WHEN THE PREGNANT PERSON IS ON PROLONGED BEDREST

Take on added responsibilities cheerfully; consider them your contribution to your baby's and the pregnant person's health and well-being. Ease your burden by getting household help, if possible. Encourage the pregnant person to shop for the baby by catalog or online. They might communicate with others on bed rest via the internet, too (see Recommended Resources, page 190). This is also a good time for them to read books and watch videos on baby care and feeding. Their childbirth educator or public library may have such videos available. YouTube and other websites also are good sources.

High Blood Pressure

About 5 percent of pregnant people have chronic high blood pressure, or hypertension, that begins either before or during pregnancy. This condition needs to be monitored carefully throughout pregnancy. Medications may be necessary, and they may need occasional adjustment.

Five to 8 percent of pregnant people develop high blood pressure (over 140/90 in two consecutive readings) after 20 weeks of pregnancy. They are said to have gestational hypertension (GH), also called pregnancy- induced hypertension (PIH), which is usually mild. Mild GH may be accompanied by swelling in the legs, hands, and face and protein in the urine. The caregiver monitors it carefully. The condition usually goes away after birth, but sometimes it becomes more severe during labor.

More severe GH, referred to by the terms preeclampsia, eclampsia, toxemia, and HELLP syndrome, can be scary. HELLP stands for hemolysis [breakdown of red blood cells], elevated liver enzymes, and low platelets. In addition to the swelling and protein in their urine, the pregnant person may have blurring or spots in their vision, upper abdominal pain, headaches, increased reflexes (that is, when the knee is tapped, the foot jerks more than usual), and liver and kidney problems (the last are detected by a blood test). The function of the placenta may be impaired, and this may slow the baby's growth. If the GH is very severe, the pregnant person may experience convulsions. Very rarely, women die from this condition. .

HOW THE PREGNANT PERSON MAY REACT
During pregnancy, the pregnant person may feel:
- Disbelief, because many people with mild, or even moderate, GH feel fine. They may not want to comply with orders to quit work or reduce activity or stay in bed. They may feel the doctor is overreacting.
- Relief, if they can quit or cut down at work, especially if it has become tiring or stressful
- Worried, when they learn some of the possible serious consequences for themselves and the baby if the condition cannot be controlled
  During labor, the pregnant person may feel:
- Disappointment over the required interventions, especially induction of labor (see page 114), restriction to bed, and electronic fetal monitoring (see page 108).
- Discomfort from the effects of medications, especially magnesium sulfate, which may make them twitch, sweat, and feel hot, flushed, and nervous. Blood pressure medications may also have uncomfortable side effects: headaches, nausea, drowsiness, shortness of breath, and trouble urinating.

HOW YOU CAN HELP
Empathize with the pregnant person and help them focus on what they must do—for their welfare and the baby's. Discuss the comfort measures they can use (see "When the Birthing Person Must Labor in Bed," page 99). Severe GH is a serious condition and requires cooperation from both of you. Remain informed of their condition, the baby's well-being, and treatments.

Gestational Diabetes Mellitus (GDM)
Gestational diabetes mellitus (GDM), also called glucose intolerance or simply gestational diabetes, first appears during pregnancy and is a potentially serious disorder regarding how the pregnant body adjusts to the increased glucose load that normally occurs in pregnancy to support fetal growth. The result is extra-high blood glucose levels in the preg-

nant person, which can increase the chances of urinary tract infections, preterm labor, a large baby, and stillbirth. The newborn is also at added risk (see folowing page). Pregnant people are offered testing around 26-68 weeks; early detection and appropriate treatment help prevent these problems.

The mainstay of treatment is a very healthy, individualized, and tightly controlled low-sugar and low-carbohydrate diet combined with regular exercise. This may be all that is necessary to keep blood sugar levels normal. If not, the pregnant person may also need to take insulin.

CONCERNS FOR THE BABY

Especially if the pregnant person's blood sugar is not well controlled, the baby's organ systems are at increased risk for uneven development because of inadequate insulin production. Effects may include:

- Large size (because of excess glucose that crosses the placenta to the baby) and associated increased risk of difficult birth
- Low blood sugar at birth due to a sudden drop in glucose from the pregnant person that occurs at birth
- Prolonged jaundice, possibly due to liver immaturity at birth
- Respiratory problems, due to developmental immaturity of the lungs, despite the baby's large size

Gestational diabetes is managed with the goal of preventing these complications. Ask the doctor about the plans for care during labor A neonatologist or pediatrician may be present at the birth to observe and care for the newborn. The prognosis for the baby is very good when the pregnant person's diabetes is well controlled.

How the Pregnant Person May React

During labor, the pregnant person may feel:

- Disbelief they are ill, especially if feeling fine
- Disappointment over the added interventions
- Worry about the baby
- Helpless or unable to understand the complexities of the treatment

HOW YOU CAN HELP

- Learn about gestational diabetes and any options the pregnant person may have (see Recommended Resources, page 190).
- Encourage the pregnant person to ask the Key Questions for Informed Decision-Making (see page 101).
- Help them understand and adjust to the demands of their diet and blood sugar testing regimen and to the necessary interventions they will experience during labor.
- Emphasize the things they can do to help themselves in labor, rather than dwelling on all the things they cannot do.

Herpes Lesion

If the pregnant person has or has ever had genital herpes, which causes sores to appear in the genital area, they should report this to the caregiver. If the virus is active when labor begins, the baby could contract the virus during vaginal birth. Though rare, herpes in the newborn is very serious; it frequently causes brain damage and death. If the herpes has been present for a long time, the risk that a sore during labor could give the baby herpes is about 1 to 3 percent; the risk is much higher if the pregnant person has recently acquired herpes.

In an effort to prevent herpes outbreaks in late pregnancy, Many caregivers offer antiviral medication (such as acyclovir or valacyclovir) during the last weeks of pregnancy to all pregnant people who have ever had herpes sores. Such treatment has resulted in a great decrease in the number of newborns who acquire the disease. A person who has not had an outbreak in years may reasonably refuse the medication, but a person who has had one or more recent outbreaks may be wise to accept it.

HOW THE PREGNANT PERSON MAY REACT

The pregnant person will probably be disappointed, shocked, angry, or depressed when learning they have an active herpes lesion, especially if it was unexpected. Expect them to need time, support, and, perhaps, counseling afterward to deal with the disappointment over any changes in plans for the birth or any problems in the baby caused by the herpes.

HOW YOU CAN HELP

- Give the pregnant person an opportunity to express their anger or disappointment.
- Give them time to adjust to the need for medications.
- Try not to become defensive if you were the source of the herpes. Your defensiveness will prolong their anger and postpone their adjustment to the cesarean.
- Explore ways to make the cesarean more satisfying (see page 155).

Excessive Bleeding During Labor

Most bleeding during labor comes from the site of the placenta, when it begins to separate from the uterine wall. The amount of visible bleeding and the seriousness of the problem depend on where and how extensive the separation is and whether the bleeding is concealed, that is, blood does not flow out. If the placenta is very low in the uterus and covers the cervix fully or partially (this condition is called placenta previa), blood comes out of the vagina. If the placenta is high in the uterus when it begins to separate (this condition is called placental abruption), the uterus may become very firm between contractions and the laboring person is in constant pain (rather than the intermittent pain that normally comes with contractions). In either case, both pregnant person and baby are in danger; potentially, this is an acute emergency.

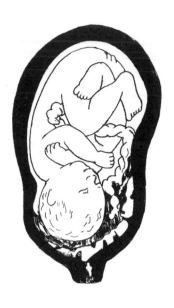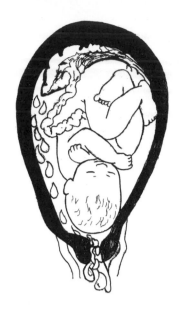

<INSERT HC8808_057.tif>

Left: placenta previa; right: placental abruption

HOW THE PREGNANT PERSON MAY REACT

During labor, the pregnant person may:

- Be caught off guard
- Be frightened for their health and the baby's health over abnormal bleeding, leaving other priorities irrelevant
- Feel very nervous about waiting and preoccupied with the baby's condition
- Wonder whether the caregiver is overreacting

HOW YOU CAN HELP

- Remain well informed about the severity of the bleeding and the baby's condition. Share the information with the pregnant person.
- Continue supporting the laboring person during contractions and remind them to deal with each contraction as it comes, not fret about what may happen.
- Be prepared to comply with changes in management and help the pregnant person comply, if the baby shows signs of distress.

Excessive Bleeding After Birth (Postpartum Hemorrhage)

Some bleeding immediately after birth is normal; it comes from the area in the uterus where the placenta was attached. The uterus usually contracts vigorously after birth, causing the bleeding to subside. You may be surprised, though, at how much blood there seems to be even under normal circumstances. Losing as much as 2 cups (475 ml) of blood is considered normal.

Postpartum hemorrhage, or excessive bleeding immediately after birth, usually occurs for one of three reasons: relaxation of the uterus, a retained placenta or fragments of placenta, or lacerations in the vagina or cervix. The loss of blood may cause the just-birthed person's blood pressure to drop; the skin may become clammy, and they may feel faint. To remedy the low blood pressure, they will be asked to lie flat, with their head low, and they will be given intravenous fluids, possibly containing a drug to raise the blood pressure.

For a few weeks after a person gives birth, they experience a dwindling discharge, called lochia. This fluid is composed of blood and some of the tissue that lined the uterus during pregnancy. Lochia is like a longer-than-usual menstrual period.

HOW THE BIRTHING PERSON MAY REACT

The birthing person may:

- Fail to realize, at first, how serious the blood loss is
- Feel weak or faint if a large amount of blood is lost
- Become frightened if bleeding continues and urgent measures are taken to stop it

Arrest of Active Labor (Dystocia)

By the time the cervix dilates to 6 centimeters, the cervix is usually quite thin and ready to open more easily. So, even if it has taken many hours, or even a day or two, to reach this point (see "The Slow-to-Start Labor," page 92), dilation now usually speeds up. Sometimes, though, it does not. Dilation may be very slow (this is called protracted labor) or it may seem to stop for 2 or more hours (this is called arrested labor).

Slow progress is not necessarily a problem, but an arrest of labor is a concern for the caregiver as well as the parents. The caregiver begins to worry that the laboring person is becoming exhausted, especially if they have tried everything and there is no end in sight. At some point, the caregiver begins to think the labor should be sped up. This is when the laboring person crosses the line from having a difficult labor, as described in chapter 5, to having a complicated labor—one requiring medical intervention.

Many things can be done to speed a prolonged labor and to support the laboring person undergoing it. You both can do some of these things (see page 96); others must be done by the nurses and caregiver.

During the prolonged labor, the caregiver may:

- Monitor the fetal heart rate more often, or continuously, to help determine whether the baby is tolerating the delay
- Offer the laboring person a narcotic or an epidural to reduce pain and help them relax, especially if they are exhausted. With an epidural or, to a lesser extent, a narcotic, they may be able to sleep, and progress may resume.
- Start intravenous fluids in the hope that improved hydration and some calories might reenergize the uterus
- Rupture the membranes in hopes of speeding labor (see page 111)

- Use intravenous oxytocin (Pitocin) to stimulate contractions if they appear to be decreasing or inadequate to change the cervix or the baby's position (see page 115)
- Use an intrauterine pressure catheter (internal electronic fetal monitoring) to find out just how strong the contractions are or whether Pitocin improves them
- Use forceps or a vacuum extractor (see pages 120–122) if the delay occurs in the birthing (second) stage
- Recommend a cesarean delivery if there is no progress even with the passage of considerable time and after efforts have been made to correct the problem (see chapter 9)

HOW THE LABORING PERSON MAY REACT

The laboring person may:
- Be willing to try suggested measures to improve progress
- Feel exhausted and discouraged if nothing seems to work
- Want a break and ask for an epidural, even if they originally wanted to avoid one (see page 147 for discussion of the code word)
- Need acknowledgment of their great efforts and validation that this labor is unusually difficult
- Fear something is wrong with their body or the fetus
- Be ready for Pitocin, a cesarean, or anything that will end the labor and bring the baby

HOW YOU CAN HELP

You can help the laboring person during an arrest of labor in these ways:
- Confer with the doula or nurse on suggestions to help the laboring person
- If the laboring person hasn't tried them yet, suggest the measures discussed in chapter 5 (see "Slow Progress in Active Labor and the Birthing Stage," page 96 and "Nipple Stimulation," pages 91–92). They may not have thought of a bath, changing positions, or labor-stimulating measures.
- If tired and discouraged, the laboring person may be reluctant to do things to make the contractions more intense. Consider their prior preferences regarding the use of pain medications (see pages 145–146). An epidural under these circumstances may allow them to sleep while the contractions intensify and (hopefully) progress to vaginal birth.
- Be attentive and understanding of the laboring person's emotional state during an exhausting labor. If they feel ignored when they express discouragement, they may later feel they were alone or unheard by you or others.

COMPLICATIONS WITH THE FETUS

The ability of the fetus to tolerate labor varies. Usually, labor benefits the baby by facilitating alertness, respiration, temperature regulation, and suckling. Sometimes, however, conditions that existed prior to labor interfere with the fetus's or newborn's well-being. The laboring person's caregiver watches for signs that the fetus is not tolerating labor well and that interventions may be needed.

PROLAPSED CORD

On very rare occasions, the umbilical cord prolapses—that is, slips below the baby into or through the cervix. This can occur before or during labor, and it is a true obstetric emergency that can result in the baby's death if not promptly and correctly managed. The danger is this: If the cord prolapses, it can be pinched by the baby's head at the cervix. This obstructs blood flow through the cord and deprives the baby of oxygen. The baby can survive only a few minutes without oxygen.

SIGNS TO RECOGNIZE

A prolapsed cord is rare under any circumstances, but is most likely to happen if two conditions are present—the baby is in a breech presentation (buttocks or feet down) or the head is high or off the cervix and the bag of waters suddenly breaks with a gush, either spontaneously or because the caregiver ruptured it. With this combination, the cord may slip down around the baby's head or buttocks as the fluid escapes; then the baby, who has been "floating," presses on the cord, slowing or stopping blood flow to the placenta and oxygen to the baby.

A cord prolapse is extremely unlikely when the baby is already low in the pelvis and the head or buttocks are already pressing against the cervix.

MANAGEMENT OF A PROLAPSED CORD

The caregiver gets the laboring person into the open knee-chest position and places a hand in the vagina to hold the baby off the cord. A cesarean section is performed as soon as possible. With this rapid action, the baby will likely be born in good health.

If you suspect there may be a cord prolapse, follow these steps:

- Call the caregiver and hospital. If you or someone else can't drive the pregnant person to the hospital immediately, call 911 and say that the pregnant person's bag of waters has broken. To ensure a rapid response, indicate there may be a prolapsed cord (even though chances are small).
- With your help, the pregnant person should get onto their hands and knees and then drop their chest down to the floor or bed. This open knee-chest position uses gravity to move the baby away from the cervix and off the cord.
- Go immediately to the hospital. Before the pregnant person stands to walk to the car,

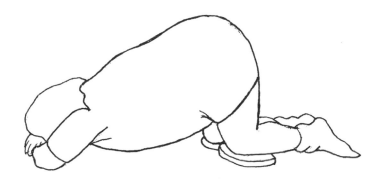

move the car close to the door of the house, move the front seat forward, and open the back door of the car for them.

- The pregnant person should ride in the back seat, or in the ambulance, in the open knee-chest position, with their buttocks high. Drive carefully, but wasting no time, to the hospital emergency entrance. Leave the laboring person in the car in the open knee-chest position. Go in and tell the person on duty that the pregnant person's bag of waters broke and you think they may have a prolapsed cord. The pregnant person should remain in the open knee-chest position on a stretcher until a doctor or nurse can listen to the fetal heart rate. If the heart rate is normal, as it most likely will be, you can all relax and rejoice. If, however, the cord had prolapsed, this could save the baby's life.

HOW YOU CAN HELP

As scary as all this is, the odds of a prolapsed cord, even if the baby is high or breech and the bag of waters breaks with a gush are low—perhaps 1 in 100. In the event of a cord prolapse, however, your and the pregnant person's actions will be most important; time and their position are the crucial factors in the baby's well-being. Cooperate with the hospital staff in whatever way possible.

Fetal Heart Rate Problems

Although a healthy baby has a remarkable ability to compensate for temporary oxygen deficits during labor, brain damage can occur if oxygen deprivation is severe and continues too long or if the baby has another problem that reduces the ability to compensate.

DIAGNOSING FETAL DISTRESS

At present, the two main indicators of fetal distress are the fetal heart rate and the presence of meconium in the amniotic fluid. See pages 108–113 for discussion of fetal monitoring and amniotic fluid characteristics.

The truth is, there is no technology that can give a clear and accurate indication of how well a baby is doing in the moment, or how likely they will do in the next hours. In a risky situation, most caregivers (and parents) are less inclined to be patient and "wait and see" whether the baby will remain stable and healthy. They are more inclined to act quickly before the condition becomes an emergency.

HOW THE LABORING PERSON MAY REACT

The laboring person is likely to react in these ways:

- Fright and shock when told the baby shows signs of fetal distress
- Accept the caregiver's decisions—no questions—under these circumstances
- After delivery, especially if it was sudden and frightening, the birthing person may have very mixed feelings: relief and joy that the baby is all right, confusion about all that happened, and regrets or doubts about the cesarean and their own behavior or decisions.

HOW YOU CAN HELP

- Keep abreast of what is going on and what staff are thinking.

- Ask questions, but do not keep the caregiver from doing what is necessary if the baby seems to be in danger.
- Ask for the quickly performed fetal scalp stimulation test (see page 111) to confirm the diagnosis of fetal distress.
- Follow the suggestions near the beginning of this chapter, keeping in mind that, if the situation is urgent, there will not be time for discussion.

COMPLICATIONS IN THE PLACENTAL STAGE

Excessive Postpartum Bleeding

Excessive bleeding during this time causes symptoms of shock in the birthing person (rapid pulse, paleness, faintness, trembling, chills, or sweating). This may be caused by poor uterine tone (uterine atony) or the uterus has stopped contracting, which is necessary to stop the bleeding. This is treated with Pitocin or other medications to make the uterus contract and stop the bleeding.

Retained Placenta

The lack of muscle tone in the uterus may prevent the birth of the placenta. Sometimes, pieces of the placenta or membranes are left behind after most of the placenta has been expelled. These fragments can also prevent the uterus from contracting fully and cause excessive bleeding. Usual treatment includes medicine to cause strong contractions, or manual removal of the placenta or fragments,

Lacerations

Sometimes, as the baby comes down the birth canal and exits the vagina, some tearing of tissues can occur and result in bleeding. Stitching (under anesthesia) is done to close the lacerations.

HOW THE BIRTHING PERSON MAY REACT

The birthing person may not be fully aware of the seriousness of the complication and may be surprised at the actions of the staff. If they have symptoms of shock from the bleeding or fear for their own well-being, they will probably be frightened, especially if you are also frightened. They will benefit from reassurance and some explanation of what is happening, especially if the caregiver will talk with them.

HOW YOU CAN HELP

Stay beside the birthing person; talk to them; and help them keep calm by breathing slowly and fully and focusing on the baby, if the baby is near or with them. Ask the caregiver or nurse to explain what is happening. If possible, encourage the birthing person to hold the baby skin to skin (with your help) and keep talking to the baby. Encourage the baby to suckle at the breast. If you are worried, sit near the birthing person and do not show your fear. Focus on the birthing person and baby at this time.

COMPLICATIONS WITH THE NEWBORN

The newborn baby is assessed immediately after birth. If all is normal, the baby is usually placed in the birthing person's arms for cuddling and suckling. If there are problems, the baby may need to go to the nursery for special care.

If the baby has problems, take part in the decision-making about appropriate care. The Key Questions for Informed Decision-Making (see page 101) will help. The birthing person may be unable to think clearly right after the birth because of the excitement and the effects of drugs, exhaustion, or problems of their own. Provided you are legal next of kin, it may fall upon you to agree to the course of treatment. (If you have no legal or biological tie to the baby—if you are, for example, a co-parent in a state where your relationship to the birthing person is not recognized or a relative or friend—make arrangements ahead of time whereby you may make decisions about the baby if the biological parent cannot.)

If the baby must remain in the special-care nursery for several days or more, you may need to be the baby's advocate, despite your distress. When a baby is hospitalized, many caregivers (for example, pediatricians, neonatologists, other physician specialists, nurses, laboratory personnel, X-ray and ultrasound technicians, respiratory or physical therapists, and social workers) are usually involved. They come and go, each providing care and information according to their roles and responsibilities. Keeping track of everything can be most confusing and may seem next to impossible. Parents and their partners often feel helpless, depressed, confused, and either distrustful of the baby's caregivers or resigned to accepting whatever they say. Good communication and record keeping are ways to prevent these feelings of helplessness.

Remain with the baby as much as possible. The baby needs a loving person close by, to hold them (if their condition permits), to stroke and talk and sing to them, and to keep track of what is going on.

When you need to leave, ask a relative or friend to stay with the baby, at least some of the time you are gone. The point is to remain informed as the various professionals participate in the baby's care.

- Keep a written log of each visit by staff, including the professional's name and specialty, date, time, purpose of the visit, and a summary of any communication regarding the baby's condition, plans for testing, medications, and so on.
- Keep all the records in one notebook, not on scraps of paper; this will make it easier for you to locate the items you want to ask about. Sometimes, there are differences in advice and contradictory information. Your notes will be most helpful as you work to keep everything straight.
- Write down your questions so you do not forget to ask them.
- Above all, know who is coordinating the baby's care and how to reach that doctor or, when off duty, a substitute.

The birthing person should remain with the baby as much as possible. Make sure they have a comfortable chair or bed and access to nourishing food. If the baby cannot breastfeed, the birthing person should be given a breast pump and instructions for using it. Pumped breast milk can usually be fed by bottle; if the baby cannot yet take a bottle, a stomach tube is used. Even if the birthing person is not planning to breast-feed, the pediatrician may ask them to provide their own colostrum or milk until the baby can take formula well, as breast milk helps protect the baby from infection during this vulnerable time. Formula cannot do this.

KANGAROO CARE

Studies show that being held skin to skin on a parent's chest and covered with a blanket keeps a baby warmer than a heated baby bed. The baby benefits not only from the parent's warmth but also from their movements, soothing voice, touch, and even heartbeat sounds. Both parent and baby are more content when they spend some hours each day in this kangaroo care.

Babies who have been "kangarooed" gain weight faster, suckle better, cry less, and are discharged from the hospital sooner. Kangaroo care has been done even with babies receiving oxygen or tube feedings or who are very premature or sick. Ask the baby's caregiver or nurse about kangaroo care and see Recommended Resources (page 190) for more information on this subject.

Detailed descriptions of all possible newborn problems are beyond the scope of this book but following are some fairly common problems that might arise shortly after birth.

Breathing Problems

A newborn may have difficulty breathing because of fluid in the lungs, meconium aspiration (see "Suctioning the Baby's Nose and Mouth," page 368), lingering narcotic drugs that were given to the birthing person during labor (see chapter 8), infection, immature lungs, or congenital abnormalities. A baby who is slow to breathe on their own, or who breathes very fast and grunts as they breathe, may need medications, intravenous feeding, an incubator, deep suctioning, resuscitation, mechanical assistance with breathing, extra oxygen, or other help.

Low Body Temperature

A baby whose body temperature drops below normal uses oxygen and energy to bring that temperature up. It is important to keep the baby warm (see "Kangaroo Care," above, and "Warming Unit," page 163).

Infection

A newborn sometimes acquires an infection while in the uterus or soon after birth. Depending on the organism causing it, the infection may be serious (see "Group B Strep Screening," page 103, or genital herpes, page 127). Prompt diagnosis and treatment with antibiotics or other medications, along with special care in the nursery (intravenous feeding, an incubator, and close observation), are needed.

Because infection in a newborn can become very serious very quickly, painful interventions may be necessary. These may include tests of various body fluids, obtained by heel sticks; spinal taps; bladder taps; scalp-vein intravenous lines; nasogastric tubes; and many other complex procedures. You and the birthing person will find all this confusing and frightening. Keep informed so you understand what is done and why and follow your baby's progress.

Birth Trauma or Injury

Some babies are injured during the birth process, especially if the birth is difficult. A very rapid birth or a prolonged or difficult forceps, vacuum, or cesarean delivery can cause bruises, a broken collarbone, cuts, or nerve damage. Although wise management reduces the chances of such injuries, they can occur even with the most skilled caregivers.

For some vulnerable babies (for example, premature babies, babies with birth defects, and babies with genetic or other preexisting problems), even the normal birth process is too much. Some very large babies also suffer, if great effort by the caregiver is required to deliver them. Vulnerable babies can usually, but not always, be identified before labor, and plans can be made in advance for their special care.

Sometimes, even with the best of care, a baby is unexpectedly born with serious problems requiring emergency treatment or long-term care. This possibility haunts parents and professionals alike and motivates attempts to develop better diagnostic and treatment methods.

Low Blood Sugar

Low blood sugar is rather common in:
- Babies of diabetic birthing persons
- Very large, small, or premature babies
- Babies whose birthing parent received large amounts of intravenous dextrose or glucose solution during labor
- Babies born after prolonged labors
- Babies born under other rare conditions, such as sepsis (infection), delayed feeding, or Rh incompatibility

Symptoms of low blood sugar in the baby include jitteriness, irritability, breathing problems, temperature problems, and others. The diagnosis of low blood sugar is made by drawing blood from the baby's heel and analyzing it. Treatment usually consists of giving the baby some glucose water or formula and rechecking blood sugar levels. The problem usually resolves itself quickly.

Jaundice

If the baby's skin or the whites of their eyes become yellowish, the baby is jaundiced. Usually harmless, physiologic jaundice is caused by elevated levels of bilirubin, a yellow pigment that results when red blood cells break down after birth as part of their normal life cycle. Physiologic jaundice is mild and goes away on its own, usually in a few days, but extra-high levels of bilirubin in some vulnerable babies may cause brain damage. Premature babies, babies who had particular difficulties during birth, and those with blood types incompatible with the gestational parent's are more vulnerable to brain damage from high bilirubin levels.

Jaundice is diagnosed by measuring bilirubin in the baby's blood, a sample of which is taken with a heel stick. Further tests of blood type, liver function, and bowel function help determine the cause of jaundice.

Jaundice is treated with phototherapy in the hospital or with portable units at home after discharge. It consists of exposing the baby's skin to special bright light almost constantly for a few days. Light breaks down bilirubin and lowers total bilirubin levels. Treatment usually lasts for a few days after which the jaundice begins to recede. Prolonged exposure to indirect sunlight (through a window) helps, but less reliably than artificial light. Frequent nursing (more than eight times per day) also helps relieve jaundice.

If bilirubin levels are very high or if the baby is premature, jaundice is more serious, and a complete exchange transfusion may be done. This is very rare today.

Death of a Baby

Rarely, a baby dies during or around the time of birth. Words cannot describe the shock and grief felt by the parents and their loved ones. Of course, nothing can bring the baby back to life, but memories can be created that will have great meaning as time passes.

As difficult as it is to think through the possibility that your baby could die, it is a good idea to learn about the kinds of things that can be done to bring some positive meaning to such a tragedy. Please see page 13 for some suggestions. Decision-making is very difficult when one is grieving intensely, but parents may later feel regret it if they did not say goodbye in the way they would have chosen. See Recommended Resources (page 190) for more helpful information.

Many hospitals have sensitive and compassionate staff members who do all they can to create a meaningful opportunity for parents to be alone with their baby. Staff members may also provide referrals for support groups and grief counseling. Please make a plan and then put it aside, with the peace of mind that you have it in case you need it. Then, focus on a healthy outcome and a beautiful baby.

AFTER IT IS ALL OVER

Any complication during labor or the early postpartum period, whether in the birthing parent or baby, presents a challenge to your family, the caregiver, the nurses, and the doula.

Each complication requires quick acceptance of a change in plans and expectations, often without a complete understanding of the situation. You do what must be done, even if in a state of shock. Afterward, as you, the parents, look back over the events, the feelings hit. Even if both birthing parent and baby have come through alive and healthy, the emotional impact can be great. Unanswered questions and feelings of guilt, anger, or disappointment may arise, especially if everything happened too quickly for either or both of you to grasp, or if you, the birthing parent, or the baby was treated unkindly or disrespectfully.

It may take time, especially for birthing parents, to come to terms with unrealized expectations. They are going through a grieving process. Your doula or a friend may be able to help with some of the practical matters, such as phone calls, lining up friends and family to help, and be a listening ear as you relive the experience with someone who was there. For both of you, a conference with the caregiver may fill gaps in your understanding of the events and answer your questions. Sometimes, consulting with a childbirth educator, trauma counselor, or psychotherapist helps either or both parents sort out feelings and gain a healthy perspective on a physically or emotionally traumatic birth experience.

CHAPTER 8

Medications for Pain During Labor

IN HOSPITAL BIRTHS, medications are also used to relieve labor pain (only nondrug remedies are used in home and birth-center births). To a great extent, drugs for pain are optional—the laboring person can decide whether and when to use them.

Because they are readily available in a variety of forms and because they can have profound effects besides pain relief, they require precautions and extra procedures for safety.

WHAT YOU BOTH NEED TO KNOW ABOUT PAIN MEDICATIONS

Find out which pain relief methods are available. The most common methods work in these ways: Narcotics or narcotic-like medications (given by pill, injection, or intravenous drip) cause sleepiness, grogginess and relaxation. Epidural and spinal blocks (given by single injection or continuous infusion into the low back near the spine) cause numbness and partial or complete inability to move the lower half of the body, but do not but have no mental effects. More rarely, general anesthesia (given by mask or injection, and used only in emergencies) makes the person unconscious. Because all pain medications involve trade-offs --possible unwanted side effects -- both the birthing person and the fetus are monitored closely so that side effects can be identified and treated quickly. Following are examples of some common side effects of various pain medications: Epidural – drop in birthing person's blood pressure; slowing of contractions; difficulty pushing during birth; malposition of the fetus; slowing of fetal heart rate. Narcotics—nausea; itching; sleepiness; inability to think clearly; inadequate pain relief. See Chapter 6 for information on problems in labor and how they are treated. You and the birthing person should discuss this topic with the care provider during prenatal appointments.

The Partner's Role When the Laboring Person Has a Narcotic

Narcotics or narcotic-like drugs require the partner's or doula's help to work well. A narcotic may help the laboring person relax between contractions but the peaks of the contractions are about as painful with the narcotic as without. A common problem is that the laboring person dozes during the early seconds of the contraction, so the peak hits them suddenly and they can't cope.

You can tell when a contraction is starting. Even if dozing, the birthing person will wince or groan before being fully aware of the contraction. Get their attention: "Okay, here it is. Open your eyes. Breathe with me. That's good." This allows them to get into a rhythm before the peak. Help them over the peak by talking and moving your hand rhythmically until they drift off again. In this way, you can maximize the benefit of the narcotic.

Regional Analgesia and Anesthesia (Epidural and Spinal)

GENERAL CHARACTERISTICS OF REGIONAL ANALGESIA

The Procedure for Giving Epidural or Spinal Analgesia (which usually takes 15 to 30 minutes)

1. Before receiving the anesthetic, the birthing person is given intravenous fluids to reduce the chance that their blood pressure will drop.
2. The birthing person lies on their side or sits up. An anesthesiologist scrubs the area where the injection will be given, numbs the skin with a local anesthetic, and then injects a small amount of anesthetic between the vertebrae of the low back (lumbar spine) (see illustrations). Sometimes, more than one attempt is needed to get the needle placed perfectly.
3. **For a spinal:** A full dose is given in a single injection that lasts 2 to 3 hours and is used for cesarean deliveries. For an epidural: A thin tube is run through the epidural needle to allow the medicine to drip in throughout the labor. Within minutes, the birthing person begins to become comfortable and numb in the desired area. Some hospitals offer patient controlled epidural analgesia, in which the birthing person can safely increase the amount of pain medicine by pushing a button. It is controlled to ensure that they don't get unsafe amounts of the medicine.
4. Once the spinal or epidural anesthetic is in place, a urinary catheter is placed in the birthing person's bladder because the birthing person is not able to urinate with the epidural in effect.

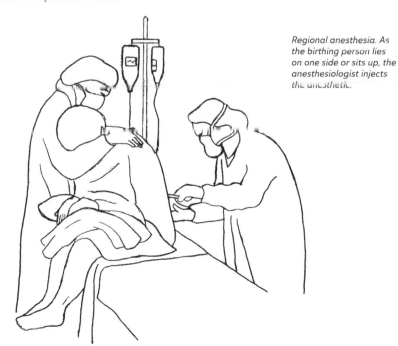

Regional anesthesia. As the birthing person lies on one side or sits up, the anesthesiologist injects the anesthetic.

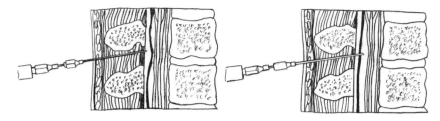

These detailed drawings illustrate the placement of the needle for an epidural block (left) and a spinal block (right)

THE PARTNER'S ROLE WHEN THE BIRTHING PERSON HAS AN EPIDURAL

An epidural usually relieves labor pain very effectively and also allows relaxation and rest or a good sleep. If labor progress is slow, the epidural makes it possible to give higher levels of Pitocin to strengthen contractions without adding pain for the birthing person. Despite the pain relief, people who have epidurals still need your companionship and help since they cannot move around very much. Once comfortable, the birthing person will no longer need intense support and close physical contact but may feel suddenly alone and unimportant if you turn on the TV, leave to get a meal, or take a nap. Unless you have a doula or other family member to remain in the room, don't leave. Continue to show support by bringing things to make them comfortable—warm blankets, ice chips, comb, toothbrush—and asking questions and making conversation. Watch TV or play a game together. Watch the monitor from time to time and point out contractions when they occur. You may both find it hard to believe that the birthing person is really having contractions, after what they have been through.

If the birthing person goes to sleep, it will likely be light and fitful. When they wake, they may feel quite alone if you are out of the room or sound asleep. If you are exhausted, of course, you may not be able to stay awake. Before you drift off, tell them to wake you if they need anything or if the doctor comes in.

- Almost forgetting they are in labor. It's easy for the birthing person to be distracted from the labor when they can no longer feel it. However, the two of you may still be able to do things to prevent some possible side effects of the epidural—slowing of labor progress and malposition of the baby. Try the six positions of the Rollover (see following), changing every 20 to 30 minutes when awake. If the nurse finds problems with any of the positions, skip it and go to the next.

Partners and the staff often believe that when the birthing person no longer has pain, they have no distress and no longer need support. Partners often take a break, get a meal, go to sleep, check their phone, get on the computer, or turn on the TV. Do not leave them unless someone remains with them.

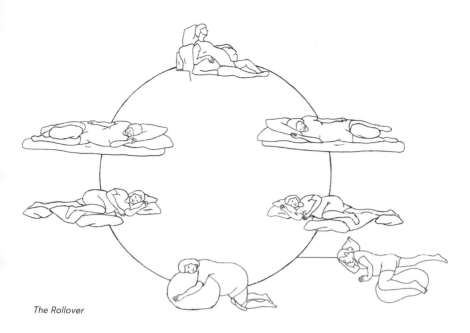

The Rollover

IF SIDE EFFECTS OCCUR

During this otherwise calm period, problems may arise that require action by the staff—for example, slowing of labor progress, a drop in the laboring person's blood pressure or the baby's heart rate, or a fever in the laboring person are all fairly common side effects of the epidural.

To speed labor, the doctor or midwife may start or increase a Pitocin (synthetic oxytocin) intravenous drip or rupture the laboring person's membranes. The nurse, watching the monitor and checking blood pressure closely, may notice the baby's heart rate slowing and have the laboring person change position and wear an oxygen mask for a while, which helps raise the baby's heart rate. If a fever occurs, the doctor or midwife may call for antibiotics because it is not possible to know whether the fever is a side effect of the epidural or due to infection. They assume it is infection , until they've tested the baby's blood.

- **Complete dilation.** You both may feel a sense of accomplishment and optimism when the cervix is completely dilated—a hurdle has been achieved! People with epidurals typically feel unable to push effectively and find it difficult to follow directions because they can't feel what they are doing. Some caregivers simply wait for up to an hour until the baby moves down and the birthing person can feel this. Then the birthing person pushes, that is, they hold their breath and strain during the contractions. Other caregivers do not wait; they want the birthing person to begin pushing as soon as they are completely dilated. Pushing is usually directed by the nurse or caregiver g—telling them when, how long, and how hard to push and when to breathe; delaying pushing until the baby is visible at the vaginal outlet or they feel the urge to push.

How you can help with pushing. When it is time to push, you or the doula can help the birthing person push well by watching the monitor for contractions, telling them when to start pushing, and cheering them on. Tell them to push when the intensity numbers go up by 20 points or so (the nurse can tell you where to look for those numbers).As the birthing person holds their breath and pushes, they make the numbers go up fast and high. You call out the increasing intensity readings from the contraction monitor to show how effective their pushing is: "20, , 40,great!. . . 60, 73, 80, 96, 100, yes! That's the way! Now, breathe for the baby . . . and bear down again. . Repeat a few times until the contraction goes away, and rest. Good! You doubled the strength of the contraction with your pushing. Great!"

This kind of encouragement the birthing person a sense of accomplishment they might not otherwise feel if they are numb. The birthing person should hold their breath for 5 to 6 seconds, which is what women do spontaneously when they do not have an epidural.

- **Rectal and vaginal pain.** As the baby's head presses on the rectum, reaches the perineum, and distends the vaginal opening, the birthing person may feel some of the same burning, stretching sensation that people without epidurals feel. This may come as an unwelcome shock after having been numb. To turn the fear to excitement, point out that the baby is almost born. If the caregiver asks the birthing person to stop pushing as the head emerges, help them pant, or "blow, blow, blow," through the contractions.
- **Vacuum extractor or forceps delivery.** This is sometimes necessary with an epidural, which may cause enough relaxation of the pelvic muscles to let the baby to descend deep in the pelvis without rotating first. The lower pelvis is smaller, which increases the chances that the baby will not rotate to fit through the pelvic outlet. If the doctor thinks an instrumental delivery may be necessary, encourage the birthing person to push as hard as they can ("give it everything you have!") to help the baby be born. It may be possible to speed the delivery and avoid the vacuum extractor or forceps and cesarean. On the other hand, it may not work, and the help of instruments may be necessary to achieve a vaginal birth.

   The birthing person may worry that the instruments will harm the baby. The doctor should describe the safety measures that protect the baby from undue force and say that, if the baby does not move with a few contractions, they will not continue with the instruments and will do a cesarean instead.
- **The birth!** The predominant emotions for the birthing person may be relief— it is over, pushing is no longer necessary—and fascination with the baby. You may have the same emotions, along with admiration and powerful love for them.

With your sensitive support, you will contribute to a safe and satisfying, though challenging birth experience

Local Anesthesia

Local anesthesia is given by injection to numb the birth canal and/or the perineum shortly before delivery (if the person does not have other anesthesia), or immediately afterwards if stitches are needed. The pudendal block numbs the vaginal canal; the perineal block numbs the perineum.

General Analgesia and Anesthesia

This form of pain-relief medication comes either as a gas to be inhaled through a mask or a mouthpiece or as a liquid injected intravenously. It reduces pain quickly by reducing or eliminating consciousness for as little as 1 minute to several hours.

INHALATION ANALGESIA: NITROUS OXIDE

Nitrous oxide mixed with oxygen (laughing gas or gas and air) is widely used in many nations for labor pain. Nitrous oxide has other uses, such as in dentistry, but it is used in stronger concentrations that would be unsuitable for labor.

Nitrous oxide is self-administered by the birthing person by inhaling the gas via a handheld mask or mouthpiece at the very beginning of (or a little before each contraction.. Within about 15 seconds, they feel drowsy, lightheaded, or giddy. As one person said, "The pain was there, but I was not bothered by it." They breathe the gas throughout the contraction, and then the mask falls away as they become less conscious. They are fully conscious by the time the next contraction comes and they inhale the gas again. In the concentrations of nitrous oxide used for childbirth today and when the birthing person holds the mask themselves, the gas wears off very quickly and effects on the baby are minimal. If someone else holds it, they may hold it on for too long, and the person may stay asleep between contractions, causing undesired side effects.

Nitrous oxide is most effective for pain in the late dilation stage, especially transition and the birthing stage. The gas is also useful in situations when quick pain relief is needed, such as manual removal of the placenta or some other painful procedure.

Nitrous oxide is considered safe for both birthing person and baby when used over a rather short time. Some side effects include nausea or vomiting 1 to 10 percent of people have nausea and vomiting,

The greatest drawback to nitrous oxide is also its greatest advantage: Its effects are immediate and very transient, lasting 1 minute or so. For women who want complete pain relief over many hours, nitrous oxide is not a good choice. But for those who want a quick assist for a few contractions or a brief painful procedure, nitrous oxide might be a good choice.

GENERAL ANESTHETICS

These systemic drugs affect the whole body. Given in the form of a gas to inhale or as an intravenous medicine, they rapidly enter the bloodstream and circulate to the brain, where they quickly abolish awareness of pain and cause loss of consciousness.

Though easy and quick to administer, general anesthetics are used rarely. There is a very small risk that the unconscious person could vomit and inhale their own vomitus, which could cause serious pneumonia. Although anesthesiologists place a tube in the birthing person's airway to prevent such a complication, general anesthesia is reserved today for the following:

- When life-threatening complications to the birthing person (such as hemorrhage) or baby (such as a prolapsed cord) require a cesarean or other surgery to be performed within minutes
- When spinal or epidural analgesia cannot be used because of specific medical conditions or anatomical anomalies in the birthing person
- When an unexpected cesarean must be performed in a hospital that does not have an anesthesiologist on duty around the clock; under such circumstances, the general anesthetic is given by the doctor doing the surgery.
- When the birthing person has expressed a strong desire to be unconscious for the birth

KNOW HOW THE BIRTHING PERSON FEELS ABOUT USING PAIN MEDICATIONS

It is important for you to know the birthing person's desires regarding the use of pain medications in labor and to explore how you feel about their use.

The Pain Medications Preference Scale (PMPS) offers the birthing person a systematic and realistic way to think about their preferred approach to pain relief and the kind of help they will need from you and others. Using the PMPS, the birthing person can state their preference about using or not using pain medications and how strongly they feel about it. You, too, should go through the PMPS to explore your own opinion and see whether you are comfortable with the birthing person's preferences.

Of course, no one knows in advance how long or painful the labor will be or whether there will be complications. A flexible approach is the only sensible one. The PMPS takes this into account by including a variety of possibilities.

After thoughtful consideration of these unknowns, the birthing person's PMPS rating will be a good predictor of whether and under what circumstances they will or will not use pain medications. The PMPS will also be a helpful guide to all who will be helping them.

Directions for Using the Pain Medications Preference Scale (PMPS)

Take plenty of time to go over the PMPS on pages 145–146. In the left column, the numbers from +10 down to +3 indicate degrees of desire to use pain medication, with +10 being the highest possible (and unrealistic) desire to use them for maximum relief of pain or any other sensations. Zero indicates no opinion. The numbers from –3 to –10 indicate degrees of desire to avoid pain medication, with –10 being an impossible extreme, just as +10 is. Everyone will be somewhere between the two extremes, which gives more meaning and clarity to the points in between.

PAIN MEDICATIONS PREFERENCE SCALE

Rating	What It Means for the Birthing Person	How a Partner and Doula Help
+10	· Desire to feel nothing; desire for anesthesia before labor begins	· An impossible extreme; if the birthing person indicates +10, help them accept that it is not possible to feel nothing in labor; the risks are too high. They will have some pain and you will help them cope. · Review the discussion of pain medications together. · Help them get pain medications as soon as possible.
+9	· Fear of pain; believes they cannot cope; dependence on staff for total pain relief	· Same as for +10, plus, · Suggest they discuss their fears with the caregiver. · Practice simple breathing and comfort techniques together. · Plan to remain with the person in labor.
+7	· Desire for anesthesia as soon as allowed or before labor becomes painful	· Same as for +9, plus, · Make sure staff are aware of their desire. Learn whether early anesthesia is possible in your hospital. · Inform staff of this desire when you arrive.
+5	· Desire for epidural anesthesia in active labor (at 5 to 6 cm, about 2 inches, dilation) · Willingness to cope until then, perhaps with narcotic medications	· Same as for +7, plus, · Encourage them in the 3 Rs (see pages 55–64). · Know comfort measures (see chapter 4) and how to help. · Suggest medications as they approach active labor.
+3	· Preference for using medication, but as little as possible, with some sensation; desire to use self-help comfort measures · Natural childbirth is not a goal.	· Same as for +5, plus, · Plan to be an active birth partner to help keep medication use low. · Help get medications when they are wanted. · Suggest low doses of narcotics or a light epidural (to allow some feeling).
0	· No opinion or preference · This attitude is rare among pregnant women, though not among birth partners or doulas.	· Make sure they are informed. · Discuss medications. · Respond to their requests in labor. · If no preference, let staff manage their pain.

PAIN MEDICATIONS PREFERENCE SCALE (CONT.)

Rating	What It Means for the Birthing Person	How a Partner and Doula Help
−3	· Wants to avoid pain medications unless coping becomes difficult · Will not feel disappointed or guilty if they use medications	· Do not suggest medications. · Emphasize coping techniques, but do not talk them out of pain medications if requested.
−5	· Strong preference to avoid pain medications, to avoid side effects for the baby or labor · Will accept medications for a long or difficult labor	· Plan to be a very active birth partner. · If possible, hire a doula to help the two of you. · Before leaving for the hospital, call and ask for a nurse who supports natural birth. · Learn and practice all the comfort measures in chapter 4 together. Know the 3 Rs (see pages 55–64). · Choose a code word (page 147) to say if they really want pain medications. Be sure staff know the code word. · During labor, do not suggest medications. · If they ask for medications, wait for the code word or have them checked for progress; try three more contractions before deciding; use the Take-Charge routine (see page 86).
−7	· Very strong desire for natural childbirth, for a sense of personal gratification as well as to benefit the baby and the progress of labor · Will be disappointed if they need to use medication	· Same as listed for −5, but with even greater commitment · Interpret requests for pain medication as a need for more help. · If they don't use the code word, keep encouraging them.
−9	· Desire that you and the staff deny the birthing person pain medication, even if requested	· Same as listed for −7 · If worried, remind them they have a code word. · Promise to help all you can but remind the birthing person that you or staff can't deny their request.
−10	· Desire that the birthing person forego all medications, even for cesarean delivery	· Impossible choice · Same as for −9: Help them develop a realistic understanding of the risks and benefits of pain medications.

After the birthing person picks the number that reflects their preferences, you should both look in the right-hand column for the kind of support and preparation needed. Can you provide this? If either of you has doubts, the birthing person can either rethink their preferences to be more in line with the kind of support you can provide, or you can get extra help from a doula or loved one. Are they preparing adequately? Make sure they understand that avoiding pain medication requires more preparation than using it.

The Birthing Person's Code Word

Many partners worry that the person who has a strong desire (-5 to -9) to avoid pain medications may, especially if labor is long or complicated, change their mind. How can you know whether it's right or wrong to keep encouraging them to continue without medications? The answer is, a code word.

You and the birthing person should agree on a word they can use if they change their mind and want pain medications. The word should be one they're unlikely to use in conversation (for example, iguana, pumpernickel, or cosmic). As long as the birthing person does not say this word, continue helping without suggesting pain medications—even if they say they want them. If they say the code word, you know they really want to change the plan, and you must respect this.

This agreement allows the birthing person to express their discouragement ("I can't do this;" "This hurts too much;" "I want drugs"), without the partner feeling a need to rescue them with medications. One doula tells of a client whose preference score was -7, but who seemed very distressed in labor. The doula said, "I was worried. I didn't want to suggest an epidural, but I was afraid she may have forgotten about her code word. So, I finally said, 'You have a code word, you know.' She never used it, so I continued to support her. Later she told me she was glad I had asked her because it made her ask herself, 'Am I suffering?' She decided she was not suffering and kept on—crying and swearing. She was glad she could complain as much as she needed to.' Complaining—always in rhythm!—was her way of coping."

CESAREAN BIRTH AND VAGINAL BIRTH AFTER CESAREAN

Sometimes, a baby is delivered surgically, through an incision in the pregnant person's abdomen, instead of through the vagina. This procedure is a cesarean section, also called a cesarean delivery, a cesarean birth, a C-section, or, simply, a cesarean. The cesarean is the most common surgery performed in the United States. The rate in 2018 was 31.9 percent, a small decline since 2009 when the rate was 32.9 percent, the highest rate ever. The causes for the high rate are numerous, complex, and controversial. In general, the attitude toward cesareans, while more accepting and unquestioning than ever before, is shifting. Recent research findings indicate long-term harm for the birthing person and baby from unneeded cesareans. See Recommended Resources (page 190) for further discussion of the cesarean rate in the United States.

Individual doctor's cesarean rates range from 10 to 60 percent of deliveries; hospitals also vary widely in their cesarean rates, from less than 10 percent to more than 65 percent in the United States.

The challenge of lowering the rate is enormous, but we are hopeful the rate will continue downward, now that the long- and short-term risks of this major surgery and its lack of benefits for healthy birthing parents and babies are becoming well known. At the same time, however, we must recognize the judicious use of the cesarean operation has, over the years, saved or improved the lives of millions of birthing persons and babies and continues to do so.

You and the pregnant person need to be able to recognize when a cesarean will improve the chances of a healthy parent and baby and when a cesarean can do more harm than good. Clear communication and covering the Key Questions for Informed Decision-Making (see page 101) with a caregiver whom you both trust, a birth setting that has a relatively low cesarean rate, and a doula are probably your most important assurances that there will not be an unnecessary or ill-advised cesarean. Numerous research studies report that birth settings in which high priorities are placed on a low cesarean rate and the presence of a doula have lower rates of cesareans and better parent and infant outcomes.

KNOW THE NONMEDICAL REASONS FOR CESAREAN BIRTH AND FACTORS TO CONSIDER

Cesareans are often done even when there is no medical reason. Among the numerous reasons are:

1. Belief that the nonmedically indicated cesarean is as safe, or safer, for the baby than vaginal birth and risks to the birthing person, though greater, are minimal. Ignorance of the risks may lead to regret over the choice.
   - Risks to the birthing persons from nonmedically indicated cesareans include surgical risks (that occur with any surgery), such as infection, hemorrhage, or bladder or bowel injury; complications in recovery; problems with incision healing; and development of abdominal adhesions, excessive internal scar tissue that binds to other structures, possibly causing chronic pain and problems with future childbearing (including more stillbirths and abnormal placental implantation). Though most people have good outcomes from cesarean deliveries, these risks should be considered, especially when there is no medical need for the surgery.
   - Risks to infants (when compared to babies born vaginally) include increased chances of serious respiratory problems; more autoimmune diseases in childhood; or more asthma, allergies, and type 1 (childhood) diabetes.
2. Deep fear of labor and vaginal birth in the birthing person (tocophobia). Every birthing person deserves education, sensitive counseling, and birth planning that addresses their fears and provides practical strategies for avoiding or minimizing those fears; these often give them the confidence to plan a vaginal birth. If, however, there is no such counseling available or they cannot come to terms with the fear, they should have the right to make the informed choice for a cesarean.

3. Fear of incontinence (involuntary loss of urine or feces) or pelvic floor damage caused by vaginal birth. These problems are rare after vaginal birth, especially with birth practices such as those discussed on pages 38–39, 40–42 and 164–165. However, they do sometimes occur in difficult vaginal births or in people with friable vaginal tissue, which is more easily injured or bleeds more easily than normal. After a few months, there is no difference in incontinence rates between those who had vaginal births and those who had cesareans. General health and fitness and body type play a greater role than mode of birth. It is true, however, that the pelvic floor is not stretched during a cesarean.

4. Convenience. The appeal for busy people and doctors of being able to plan the date and time for a cesarean is great—especially if they think the risks are acceptable. While it is undeniably more convenient for doctors, women should weigh the potential risks to themselves and their babies against this benefit, as the prolonged recovery time may negate the convenience of planning the date.

KNOW THE MEDICAL REASONS FOR CESAREAN BIRTH

You and the birthing person should understand the reasons for the cesarean before it is done and agree it is the right thing to do. If you find out in advance that the birthing person or the baby has a medical problem requiring a cesarean delivery or making it highly likely, you both can learn all about the surgery and adjust emotionally beforehand. If the need for the cesarean arises in labor, you both will have to do much of the adjusting afterward. Either way, the birthing person should have the opportunity to talk about the experience with you, your doula, the doctor, and the nurses.

See chapters 6 and 7 for information about problems that sometimes arise in labor and how they are detected and treated; a cesarean becomes the solution if other treatments are unsuccessful.

Following are the most likely medical reasons for a cesarean. Although cesareans are not always necessary in these circumstances, they are always considered and very often done.

1. Preexisting conditions that lead to planning a cesarean in advance. Most cesareans are unplanned and the need becomes clear once labor is underway. There are, however, some situations better handled by planning a cesarean for a few days before the due date. For example, some chronic illnesses or conditions: heart disease; some cases of diabetes; asthma; physical disability; some cases of twins or triplets; fetal growth restriction; placenta previa; breech presentation; deep fear of vaginal birth; previous cesarean delivery; and others. While some of these are controversial, they are among the labors considered to be at higher risk and more unpredictable than when these conditions do not exist. Parents should ask the key questions (see page 101).

If a decision is made to have a planned cesarean, read this chapter because planned and unplanned cesareans have much in common. The one bit of advice we want to add is, when setting the date and time for a planned cesarean, try to schedule it early or as the first case of the day, for two reasons: It is less likely to be a delayed (from earlier surgeries taking longer than expected) and the birthing person will likely be instructed to eat nothing after midnight; if they do not have to wait until late in the day, they'll be much more comfortable.

2. Emergencies that arise in labor, including:
- Prolapsed cord (see page 131)
- Serious hemorrhage (excessive bleeding) in the birthing person (see page 128); in these situations, there is no time for questions. Rapid action is essential.

3. Arrested labor. This is the most common reason for a first cesarean. Failure to progress in labor may be caused by the following:
- Abnormal position or presentation of the baby
- Uterine inertia (inadequate contractions)
- A poor fit between the baby's head and the birthing person's pelvis
- A combination of more than one of the above indications

According to many experts, far too many cesareans are performed because of arrested labor, or "failure to progress." Many of these cesareans are done for failure to *wait* rather than failure to progress. In fact, the American College of Obstetricians and Gynecologists has recently published several documents offering evidence-based guidelines for reducing primary (first) and repeat cesareans (see Recommended Resources, page 190).

4. Problems with the fetus, including:
- Fetal intolerance of labor. Many experts believe this is another reason for which cesareans are too often performed (see "Diagnosing Fetal Distress," page 132).
- Breech presentation
- Prematurity, postmaturity (when the baby is overdue), or other conditions that might make vaginal birth too stressful for the baby. Through fetal movement counting, by which the birthing person keeps track of how much the baby moves (see page 188), nonstress testing (see page 104), and ultrasound (see page 104), the caregiver tries to predict whether the baby can tolerate labor.

5. Problems with the birthing person, including:
- Serious illness (such as heart disease, diabetes, or preeclampsia) or injury. Sometimes, in these cases, a cesarean is planned in advance. Otherwise, a "trial of labor" is planned. The birthing person is watched carefully and, if all goes well, they give birth vaginally. If the problem worsens, they have a cesarean.
- A genital herpes sore (see page 127)

6. A previous cesarean delivery. This is a major reason for the high cesarean rate in the United States and Canada. Today, approximately 87 percent of people who have had a cesarean will have another, even though most are good candidates for a VBAC. With the right doctor and hospital, a VBAC is possible. Furthermore, there is good reason to believe that VBACs will increase now that ACOG and other professional organizations strongly support VBACs under safe conditions.

Once the decision to perform a cesarean is made, concentrate on helping the birthing person and greeting the baby as lovingly and gently as possible.

KNOW WHAT TO EXPECT DURING CESAREAN BIRTH

You may be surprised by how quickly the staff move once the decision is made to do a cesarean and by the number of people involved: Besides you, possibly a doula, and the birthing person, there is the doctor who will do the surgery; an assisting doctor or midwife; a "scrub nurse," who gives instruments to the doctor; a "floating nurse," who prepares the room and looks after the surgical team; an anesthesiologist; a pediatric nurse or two to look after the baby; and possibly a pediatrician or neonatologist, if problems with the baby are anticipated. They all work together as an efficient, businesslike team.

You may feel frightened and worried for the birthing person or baby. You may feel relieved to know the end is in sight, especially after a long, difficult labor. You may be impressed and reassured by the teamwork and competence of the staff. You may feel left out or even shocked by their apparently casual attitude. They may talk and even joke among themselves, paying little attention to you and the birthing person, as if you are not there. You may feel overwhelmed by the sounds, smells, and sights of the operating room. You may be confused about your role. Should you ask questions and try to make sure the birthing person's wishes are being followed, or should you stay out of the way and let them proceed in their customary manner? Just a few minutes before, your role was essential to the birthing person's ability to handle the contractions; now you feel much less important. Be assured: you are still most important, but in a different way. The following descriptions of the surgery and your role will help you help the laboring person.

Preparations for Surgery

Preparations for cesarean delivery include the following steps:

- The birthing person signs a consent form.
- A nurse starts intravenous fluids in the birthing person's arm, which is placed on a board that extends out to the side of the operating table. The nurse checks the birthing person's blood pressure frequently.
- An anesthesiologist, nurse-anesthetist, or, rarely, the obstetrician gives the anesthetic (spinal, epidural, or general; see chapter 8). The choice of anesthesia depends on the birthing person's situation, training and qualifications of the staff, and the facilities. General anesthesia, being fastest, is chosen if the cesarean must be done immediately—which is very rare. Regional anesthesia is safer if time allows.
- The birthing person will probably receive oxygen, administered with a face mask or nasal prongs (tubes that blow oxygen into the nose).

- A pulse oximeter, a small device that tracks the oxygen content in the birthing person's blood, will be clipped to a finger or toe.
- Electrocardiogram (EKG or ECG) leads are placed on the chest. These keep track of the birthing person's heart function throughout the surgery.
- The birthing person's abdomen is scrubbed. Some pubic hair may be removed.
- A catheter is placed in the bladder to keep it empty and out of the way of the scalpel (surgical knife).
- The birthing person's body is draped so only the abdomen can be seen. The end of the drape is raised to form a screen between their head and abdomen. Even if conscious, the birthing person cannot see the surgery. Although some hospitals have a clear window in the drape so the birthing person can see the baby being lifted from their abdomen.
- Most hospitals now welcome the birth partner (and sometimes a doula or other person) in the operating room for a cesarean. You sit on a stool at the head. The anesthesiologist remains at the head also.
- Some birth partners want to watch and even photograph the surgery. Discuss this option with the birthing person and the caregiver, if it interests you both. It is quite likely for staff to refuse to let you photograph the surgery, but you can photograph the baby's first contact with their gestational parent and other tender moments. To see or photograph the baby's birth, you will have to stand up and look over the drape or hold your camera high. Try asking the anesthesiologist to take pictures; they're often happy to oblige.
- The birthing person's abdomen is scrubbed in preparation of the surgery.

Surgery Begins

This is how a cesarean delivery starts:

- Once the anesthetic takes effect, the doctor makes the incisions with a scalpel.
- The skin incision is usually low and horizontal, or transverse (this is called a "bikini incision" meaning it is so low that later, even when one wears a bikini, the scar will not be visible). Rarely, the incision is vertical and in the mid-abdomen (called a classical incision).
- The muscles of the abdomen are not cut; there is a connective tissue line (the "linea alba") down the middle of the abdominal muscles. These often separate spontaneously and painlessly during late pregnancy, as the muscles stretch around the growing uterus. During the cesarean, the surgeon spreads the muscles further, without cutting them. The incision in the uterus is made through the gap between those muscles.
- The uterine incision is usually horizontal, or transverse, in the lower segment of the uterus, but it can be made higher if speed is essential or if the higher opening is needed to get the baby out (for example, in the case of twins, a premature baby, or an unusual presentation).
- The amniotic fluid is suctioned from the uterus with a plastic tube. You will hear the sucking sound.

- To prevent excessive bleeding, the cut blood vessels are cauterized. You may hear the high-pitched tone of the cautery device or notice a slight odor as it heats the ends of the blood vessels to close them. The birthing person cannot feel this.
- If at any time during the procedure the birthing person indicates they feel pain (as opposed to pressure or tugging), make sure the doctor knows it and stops working until more anesthetic can be given. This does not happen often, but sometimes the anesthesia is spotty and the birthing person is not numb where they need to be.

The Baby Is Born!

The baby is usually delivered within 15–30 minutes after surgery has begun. This is how:

- The doctor either places one hand in the uterus to grasp the baby's head or buttocks or may instead attach a vacuum extractor to the baby's head if it is accessible (vacuum extraction allows for a smaller incision in the birthing person's abdomen). The assisting doctor pushes on the birthing person's abdomen to move the baby down to the incision. The first doctor removes the baby. The birthing person may feel pressure and tugging, but should not feel pain. Help them use relaxation and slow rhythmic breathing (see page 61). Make sure the doctor and anesthesiologist know if they complain of pain, so more anesthetic can be given.
- The doctor or nurse suctions the baby's airways and clamps and cuts the cord. You may want to ask the doctor to lower the drape so the birthing person can see the baby, or the baby may be briefly held up for you both to admire. Then, the baby is usually taken to an infant care area in the corner of the delivery room or in an adjacent room, for evaluation and any necessary treatment. By this time, the baby is probably crying lustily. You may wish to go look at and greet the baby, especially if your doula can remain with the birthing person. This is a nice time to talk with the baby, sing to them, and welcome them to the world.
- The oxygen apparatus is removed from the birthing person's face.

In some hospitals, some caregivers now delay clamping and cutting the umbilical cord for a short time or "milk" the cord to allow some placental blood to return to the baby.

Some hospitals have adopted practices (sometimes referred to as the natural or gentle cesarean), that keep the baby and birthing parent together skin to skin, starting right after the cesarean or shortly after a brief observation in the infant care unit located in or close to the operating room. They value the practice of placing the unwrapped baby on the birthing person's bare chest and then covering the baby (see page 135).

If so, the birthing person might be trembling and feel weak, so help them hold the baby on the chest, and you both can sing your baby's song or talk to the baby. These practices that encourage parent- baby contact from birth have the advantages of keeping the baby warm and enhancing bonding, feeding, and breast-seeking behaviors, Furthermore, skin-to-skin contact early after birth, enhances the birthing person's and baby's own production of oxytocin (the "love hormone").

The Placenta Is Removed

While you are greeting the baby, the doctor reaches into the uterus, separates the placenta from the wall of the uterus, and removes it.

Some doctors then lift the uterus out of the abdomen to check it thoroughly before beginning to close the incision. The birthing person may feel this as uncomfortable pressure and may feel nauseated and vomit, turning their head to the side and using the basin that you, the doula, or the anesthesiologist holds for them. Because the benefit of removing the uterus is questionable and because it causes the birthing person much discomfort (even with anesthesia), many physicians have safely discontinued the practice. Others believe it is the only way they can repair it well. You might discuss this with the doctor ahead of time, and the birthing person might state in the birth plan that they prefer not to have the uterus lifted out for inspection.

The Repair Begins

The repair phase takes 30 to 45 minutes. These procedures are involved:

- The uterus and other internal layers are sutured with absorbable suture thread. You might ask ahead of time whether the caregiver does a single-layer or double-layer repair of the uterine incision. Some doctors use the single-layer repair because it is quicker, but studies have found that single layer suturing leaves the uterine scar weaker and more likely to separate in a future pregnancy or labor. Consider asking for a double-layer repair in the birth plan.
- The skin is closed with stitches or, less frequently, stainless steel clips. You may hear the clicking of the stapler as the clips are placed.
- A bandage is applied over the incision.
- The birthing person may be very shaky, trembling all over, or nauseated— normal reactions after major surgery—so they might be given a relaxing, sleep-inducing medication via the intravenous line, without either of you knowing it. If it is important to the birthing person to be awake after the birth to experience the first hours with the baby, ask ahead of time and again just after the birth, that these medications not be given without first checking with the birthing person. The nausea and trembling usually subside within 30 minutes. If the nausea and trembling are extreme, the birthing person can always change their mind and ask for medication. It takes effect within 2 minutes.

  There is one medication, Versed, that the birthing person should be warned about. Along with being an effective sedative, it is also a potent amnesiac. It wipes out all memory of the birth and related events for hours afterward. The birthing person will not remember having the baby, nor will they remember their first impressions or the first feeding. The absence of memory of the momentous event might haunt them and cause much regret later.

  Zofran is an effective antinausea medication that does not make a person groggy or take away their memory. Ask about it or other medications that do not cause drowsiness.
- The birthing person is cleaned and taken to the recovery area.

The Recovery Period

This is what you can expect during the recovery period:

- The birthing person remains in the recovery room or in the labor room for a few hours with a nurse close by, until it is clear the recovery is going well and the anesthetic is wearing off as expected.
- The nurse frequently checks the birthing person's pulse, temperature, blood pressure, uterine tone, and state of anesthesia.
- The baby may remain with their parents or go to the nursery for observation or treatment, depending on the baby's condition and hospital custom. You might go with the baby; it is very helpful if the birthing person has the company of a friend, relative, or doula if you leave.
- A pain medication regimen will be established to keep the birthing person comfortable.
- If they haven't already done so in the operating room, the birthing person can breastfeed the baby now. The nurses or doula can help position the baby and get started. It is a good idea to begin breastfeeding before the anesthesia wears off, as it will be a little easier to get started when not in pain.
- If the birthing person is asleep or groggy from the medication for nausea and trembling, it will be difficult to breastfeed. This is why some people refuse medication for nausea and trembling, preferring to put up with it for 30 minutes to 1 hour—they do not want to miss the first few hours with the baby.
- If the birthing person is unable to nurse or hold the baby, you do it. Hold the baby close (skin to skin, if possible) and talk or sing to them.
- The nurse checks the baby's breathing, skin color, temperature, and heart rate frequently.
- Once the anesthesia wears off and the birthing person's condition is stable, they will go to the postpartum room, where they will stay until they go home. See chapter 10 for information about the first few days after birth.

YOUR ROLE DURING AND AFTER A CESAREAN BIRTH

For one who plans a vaginal birth, a cesarean is unexpected and may be disappointing, even if they know the surgery has made it possible to have a healthy baby. Some get over these feelings quickly; others do not. A birthing person often needs time afterward to adjust emotionally, to talk about and even grieve over the experience, especially if they had a strong desire to give birth vaginally. It is sometimes surprising to loved ones, nurses, and caregivers how deeply disappointed some people are and how much patience and understanding they may need from loved ones, the doula, and staff to come to terms with their baby's cesarean birth.

They are less likely to grieve for a long time if they have been able to participate thoroughly in the labor and in the decision to have a cesarean. Prolonged anger, depression, or guilt may result if the birthing person was caught by surprise and could do nothing or if they did not understand the need for it. How you respond to the birthing person's worries and feelings, both during and after the cesarean, can make a big difference in how well they adjust. Here are guidelines:

- Your perceptions of what happened will be very important to the birthing person as they put the pieces together. Try to stay with them during surgery, hold their hand, and talk to them. They may want you to take pictures, especially after the baby is born; check with staff before doing so. Many people, especially if unaware during and after the surgery, treasure such photographs later; the photos help fill in the parts they missed. It is quite likely that staff will not okay photos during the actual surgery, citing legal concerns. However, early pictures of the baby and the first feedings will be treasured.

- The birthing person will probably feel some discomfort during surgery. If it is painful, not just pressure or tugging, ask for more anesthetic to be given. You should help them focus on relaxing and breathing in a slow rhythm to handle the anxiety and sensations of pressure and tugging.

- After the birth, you will probably be able to get close to the baby and to get a good look, see, touch, stroke, talk to, and sing to the baby. The thought of talking or singing to the baby in the operating room may seem strange, but, if you are the baby's parent or the birthing person's spouse, the baby knows your voice and will respond when hearing it. You may be able to soothe the baby as no one else can besides the birthing person.

  Think of this birth from the baby's point of view—an abrupt tug out of the warm and familiar womb to a bright, cold, noisy place. They are handled competently but perfunctorily and hear only strangers' voices. Then, you come close and say, "Hi, Baby! I'm so glad to see you. Everything is all right, and I'm here to take care of you." Or, you sing a song, perhaps the one you sang aloud often during the pregnancy. You stroke the baby's arm and put your finger into the palm of their hand. The baby stares into your eyes and clings to your finger. At last, a familiar voice and loving touch for the baby! You will always cherish this moment.

- As we said earlier, it may be possible for the baby to go straight to the birthing person. If the baby goes first, though, to the infant warmer for examination, you might go there, too; bring the baby to the birthing person as soon as possible, so they can see, touch, and kiss the baby.

- Help the birthing person breast-feed or chest-feed in the recovery room. They may need your help holding the baby to the breast.

  If the baby must go to the nursery for special care, you may want to go along to see for yourself what is being done and fill in these gaps for the birthing person later. Or, you can stay with the birthing person, to give comfort and ease your own worries about their well-being. This is a difficult choice. If a family member or doula can stay with one, then you can be with the other and have some peace of mind.

- Physical recovery from a cesarean can take weeks or months. Pain, weakness, and fatigue are great at first, and the birthing person may require narcotics or other pain medication (injections, pills, or IV) for days or longer. It may take weeks or months for the last step—from functioning fairly well to returning to their pre-pregnant condition. Encourage them to rest and focus on feeding the baby while you take over the housework or get help from others. Many new parents enlist the help of friends and family or postpartum doula to provide meals, run errands, do household chores, and help with baby care and feedings.

- It may take the birthing person longer to recover emotionally than it takes to recover physically. Be patient. Give them time and fill in any gaps in their memory or understanding of what happened and why.

People vary in how long it takes them to integrate and accept the cesarean birth experience. For some, a cesarean is a positive experience; for others it is not. If the birthing person is disappointed, accept their feelings as valid and normal. Too often the birthing person's loved ones try to distract them from thinking about the birth by pointing out "all that matters" is the baby is healthy—but that is not all that matters. How one gives birth also matters, and their loved ones' patience, acceptance, and concern for these feelings will help the birthing person work through them.

- If the birth experience was particularly negative or traumatic for the birthing person, they may benefit from professional counseling or therapy. Call the caregiver or childbirth educator or doula for referrals, see Recommended Resources (page 190).
- See chapter 7 for more suggestions about the birth partner's role when problems arise during labor.

Despite feeling possible disappointment with the birth experience and the slower recovery, which is usual after a cesarean, it is unlikely that the birthing person will extend that disappointment to the baby. A cesarean birth is, after all, a birth, and all the emotions that come with birth and meeting one's baby also come with cesarean birth. The birthing person's ability to love, feed, enjoy, and care for the baby are not altered by the fact that the baby was born by cesarean. Enjoy this child together.

CHAPTER 9

The First Days Postpartum

DURING THE FIRST FEW DAYS AFTER THE BIRTH, there is much going on physically, medically, and emotionally with both the birthing parent and the baby. This chapter explains what to expect—what the caregiver does, some important choices, and your role in all this. Your primary duty, of course, is to stay with your family and give them as much emotional support and practical help as possible.

THE FIRST FEW HOURS

Immediately after the birth, the baby's well-being is quickly assessed. The nurse or midwife checks the baby's Apgar score, temperature, pulse and respiration, state of alertness, and general behavior (see page 51). Assuming all is well, the baby is dried and placed naked on the birthing parent's chest. Both are covered with warm blankets. This skin-to-skin contact is really the best way to keep the baby warm—better than wrapping or placing the baby under warming lights. It is also the perfect setting for beginning life outside the womb. The birthing parent's smell, voice, warmth, touch, and heartbeat provide familiarity and a gradualness to the baby's adjustment. The baby is also giving important gifts to the parents. When the baby is alert and staring into the parents' eyes—they can't take their eyes off each other— they're falling in love! The baby's wiggling squirming limbs massage the soft warm abdomen of the birthing parent, stimulating the uterus to contract and aiding the birthing parent's first steps in recovery.

The baby's nuzzling at the breasts also helps the uterus contract and initiates the process that ends with the baby grasping the birthing parent's nipple and suckling vigorously. As parents, you will likely be focused completely on the baby—except when reality reenters in the form of the caregiver or nurse's necessary intrusions. Their agenda is different from yours: Their main concern is the physical well-being of the birthing person and baby. So, while the two of you are engrossed in the baby, they are dealing with the following immediate clinical concerns.

Care of the Birthing Parent's Perineum

After a vaginal birth, the caregiver carefully inspects the vagina and perineum to determine whether stitches are necessary. This examination is often somewhat painful if there has been no anesthesia. An episiotomy (see page 118) or a sizeable tear will require stitches. If needed, and the birthing parent is not already anesthetized, the caregiver places a local anesthetic in the perineum. The stitches will be gradually absorbed as the incision heals; they do not have to be removed. An ice pack applied to the perineum now brings great relief.

Care After a Cesarean Birth

Following a cesarean birth (described in chapter 9), the birthing parent leaves the operating room and spends a few hours in a recovery room or labor room while the anesthetic wears off. They may be very sleepy, depending on the drugs given. There will be a nurse close by all the time. You can remain with the birthing person and, unless the baby has a problem that requires care in the nursery, the baby will be with you, too. If the baby is in the nursery, you may be with the baby or the birthing parent—a tough choice. A family member or friend could remain with the birthing person so you could go to the nursery, or vice versa.

The Vital Signs of Birthing Parent and Baby

The caregiver frequently checks the vital signs (pulse, respiration, temperature, and blood pressure) of the birthing parent and baby and performs other routine assessments. If either the birthing parent or baby had medical problems during the pregnancy or labor, the nurse or caregiver watches even more closely. They will also check the birthing parent's lochia (see page 127).

The Birthing Parent's Uterus

The nurse checks the uterus frequently to make sure it is contracting firmly. If it is soft and relaxed, it will bleed too much. It usually contracts well on its own, but, if not, there are three ways to cause it to contract:

1. Nipple stimulation: When the baby suckles at the breast, the hormone oxytocin is released, which makes the uterus contract. If the baby is not ready for a feeding, you or the birthing parent can stroke or roll their nipples, which has a similar effect.

2. **Fundal massage:** The nurse or midwife does this, but the birthing parent can learn to do it, too. This massage involves firmly kneading the low abdomen until the uterus contracts (they can feel it becoming firm as they massage it) to the size and consistency of a large grapefruit. This is painful for the birthing parent, which is one reason they may want to do it; they can do it less vigorously and get the same results.

3. **Injection or intravenous administration of Pitocin or another uterine stimulant:** This is often done routinely as the baby is being born, but may also be done later, if necessary. This is the most reliable way to contract the uterus; it may be used along with the methods described previously, although it is not needed in most cases.

Placental Encapsulation

A growing trend among pregnant and postpartum families is to have the placenta prepared and encapsulated for consumption after the baby is born. There are numerous ways to prepare the placenta, but most include steaming, dehydrating, pulverizing the desiccated placenta into powder, and placing the powder into capsules for consumption. The thought is that consuming the placenta, rich in iron and hormones, imparts many health benefits such as minimizing postpartum depression, providing additional energy, and increasing milk supply. It is important to know there is scant scientific evidence to support these claims, though there are numerous positive personal stories from parents who have tried it. There are currently studies underway to investigate the composition of desiccated placenta powder, as well as at least one carefully controlled scientific trial comparing possible benefits and risks of consuming capsules containing placenta with placebo-filled capsules during the postpartum period.

If having the placenta encapsulated appeals to you and the birthing parent, you can either search online for ways of preparing it yourselves, or you can hire a placenta encapsulation specialist to do this for you. The cost varies from about $150 to $500 depending on experience and where you live. When selecting someone to prepare the placenta, ask about their experience and training, safety protocols, where the placenta will be prepared (in your home or their preparation space), the preparation method used, and how their equipment is cleaned (see Recommended Resources, page 190).

There are some circumstances under which it is not considered safe to encapsulate the placenta. If the placenta cannot be properly refrigerated or kept cool following the birth or if it has been refrigerated longer than 4 days, it should not be encapsulated. If you were diagnosed with chorioamnionitis (infection of the bag of waters) or if your placenta needed to be sent to the hospital pathology department for testing, it is not considered safe to encapsulate. Finally, if you have a blood-borne pathogen such as hepatitis or HIV/AIDS, the hospital will generally not release the placenta for preparation. Some placenta specialists have additional contraindications such as Group B streptococcus or meconium staining of the amniotic fluid. Discuss these scenarios with your specialist. It bears repeating: there is no scientific evidence to support the claims of placenta encapsulation. However, at the time of writing, studies are underway.

Common Procedures in Newborn Care

In the first few minutes or hours after birth, the baby is examined and a number of procedures are done. Many of these are routine; others are optional. Some are required by law to detect or prevent certain serious conditions. Because the birthing parent may be exhausted or preoccupied with the procedures they are still undergoing, it will be up to you to keep track of what is happening to the baby, remind staff of the birthing parent's preferences regarding newborn care, and help the birthing parent make decisions, if necessary.

SUCTIONING THE BABY'S NOSE AND MOUTH

The baby's airway may contain mucus, amniotic fluid with or without meconium, or blood. There are two ways to deal with this fluid: the caregiver observes the baby and suctions only if the baby is not breathing or is not vigorous. It may also be done routinely—the caregiver inserts the tip of a rubber bulb syringe several times into the baby's nostrils and mouth and suctions the secretions out.

Sometimes, if the amniotic fluid was stained with meconium, deeper suctioning is done via a long tube passed through a nostril and down the baby's trachea (windpipe).

Purposes of suctioning: Suctioning is done to clear the airway of secretions, especially if the baby is unable to cough or sneeze to remove them, or to assist a baby who is not breathing. It is done routinely in many hospitals, but they are not practicing according to up-to-date scientific evidence. When a baby can breathe, suctioning is unnecessary because the baby is fully capable of coughing or sneezing the fluids out. The American Academy of Pediatrics recommends reserving any type of suctioning only for babies who have obvious obstruction and cannot breathe, or who require positive pressure ventilation (mechanically assisted respiration).

Disadvantages of suctioning: The baby may experience brief discomfort and stress and may gag, flinch, or struggle or possible abrasions of the mucous membranes in the baby's nose and throat may occur if the tip scrapes them.

Alternatives to consider: Parents can ask the caregiver to withhold suctioning of the mouth, nose, and throat unless the baby is unable to rid their airway of secretions. If suctioning is necessary, the caregiver can use the syringe gently.

CUTTING THE UMBILICAL CORD

Once the baby is out, the cord is clamped in two places and cut with scissors. You might wish to cut the cord. The nurse will give you the scissors and show you exactly where to cut.

Pros and cons of early versus late clamping and cutting the umbilical cord: Until recently, the custom was to clamp and cut the cord immediately after birth—for efficiency and to enable removal of the baby from the birthing parent to a newborn unit where the baby could be assessed and given the initial procedures (described in these pages). It was believed that early cord clamping prevented newborn jaundice. This practice came into question when research studies comparing early and late cord clamping found that the likelihood of jaundice does not increase with late cord clamping.

Studies have also found that the baby benefits from delaying cord clamping in many ways:

1. Because the size of the placenta diminishes as the blood drains from it into the baby, delivery of the placenta occurs sooner.
2. The baby continues to receive oxygen from the blood in the cord until the cord stops pulsating—especially helpful for babies who are slow to start breathing.
3. The increased volume of blood circulating to the baby's lungs hastens optimal respiration.
4. The baby's iron stores increase by as much as 45 percent, and anemia is less likely to occur in the baby for as long as 6 months.
5. Premature babies are less likely to require blood transfusions (see Recommended Resources, page 190).

All this occurs because the blood in the placenta is the baby's blood and amounts to approximately 150 milliliters (5 fluid ounces; about one-third of the baby's total blood volume). Until the cord is clamped or stops pulsating, this blood is transferred from the placenta to the baby. The best way to make sure the baby has its full allotment of blood is to place the baby on the birthing person's belly and wait for the cord to stop pulsating.

An exception to delaying cord cutting is when the baby is very ill and needs immediate medical attention (because of prematurity, breathing in large amounts of meconium, or a low Apgar score; see page 106). Then, the baby is removed to a resuscitation bed.

EYE MEDICATION

An antibiotic (usually erythromycin ointment) is placed in the baby's eyes within the first hour after birth.

Purposes of eye medication: The antibiotic prevents serious eye infection or even blindness due to the bacteria that cause gonorrhea or chlamydia—two common sexually transmitted diseases. These bacteria are sometimes present in the vagina and can be transmitted to the baby during birth.

Eye medication is medically indicated if the birthing parent tests positive for chlamydia or gonorrhea or if either parent may have been exposed to the diseases (via sexual contact with someone who has the disease). Because the lab tests are not 100 percent reliable and the organisms can appear if sexual contact occurred after the lab tests were done, the eye medication is required by all states and provinces.

Disadvantages of eye medication: The medicine blurs the baby's vision for a short time, until the warmth of the baby's eyes melts the ointment.

A very popular alternative is to ask the nurse or midwife to postpone putting the ointment in the baby's eyes until an hour or two after birth, so the baby will be able to see your faces clearly in the meantime.

VITAMIN K

Required in most U.S. states and Canadian provinces, vitamin K is given as an injection shortly after birth. This vitamin is essential in blood clotting. Newborns are relatively slow in clotting their blood for the first week or so, although once they start consuming and digesting colostrum and milk, they begin making their own vitamin K. Until then, they are at a very small risk for excessive bleeding (called vitamin K deficiency bleeding, or VKDB). Giving vitamin K to tide them over reduces the risk of bleeding problems.

Until recently, vitamin K was sometimes given by mouth, but it was found that oral vitamin K does not prevent later onset of VKDB, so the American Academy of Pediatrics now recommends only injectable vitamin K, although they call for more research on the oral form. The injection is given once, in the thigh, within an hour after birth.

Purposes of giving vitamin K: The injection is quick, easy, and inexpensive and is very effective in preventing VKDB. Giving vitamin K is especially important when a baby is at greater risk of bleeding, for example, after a difficult or instrumental birth, prematurity, or plans for circumcision before the baby is 1 week old.

Disadvantages of giving vitamin K: The injection is briefly painful. The safety of the low dose given to newborns is well established.

Alternatives to consider: Refusing vitamin K altogether is a somewhat risky option because it is not possible to predict which babies will or will not develop this rare condition—vitamin K deficiency bleeding (VKDB).

BLOOD TESTS

Virtually every newborn has at least two blood tests in the first two days. Blood samples are obtained in two ways:

1. A few drops of the baby's blood are drawn from the heel or a vein to check for:
   - Bilirubin levels, a yellowish blood pigment that, at high levels, causes jaundice (see page 136)
   - Blood sugar (glucose) levels
   - Infection, if the birthing parent had a fever in labor or if the baby has one now
   - Numerous genetic or congenital disorders (see "Newborn Screening Tests," page 166)
2. Blood from the baby's umbilical cord may also be collected at birth for:
   - Blood typing
   - Rh determination
   - Storage or donation to a blood bank (see page 366 and Recommended Resources, page 190)

Purposes of blood tests: The general purpose of testing the newborn's blood is to record the baby's blood type and detect rare but potentially serious problems early enough to treat them and prevent dangerous effects on the baby. Tests for congenital disorders are mandated by state laws. Early identification of many congenital disorders often means early treatment with very good outcomes. Without treatment, some disorders become increasingly severe and disabling for the child.

Disadvantages of blood tests: The heel stick is briefly painful to the baby, and some of the tests (such as those for bilirubin and blood glucose) may have to be repeated several times because blood levels can change over time.

Also, results of some blood tests are sometimes confusing and can lead to overtreatment. Caregivers sometimes disagree on when bilirubin and blood glucose levels require treatment. Ask the key questions (see page 101) to learn enough to make an informed decision about any recommended tests.

Alternatives to consider: You and the birthing parent can ask the caregiver about less painful ways to gain the information provided by the blood tests.

WARMING UNIT

A warming unit is a special bed with a heater above it. A baby placed in a warming unit has a small thermostat taped to the abdomen; the thermostat automatically turns up the heat if the baby becomes chilled. Small or premature babies become chilled more easily than average-size or full-term babies.

Purpose of the warming unit: The unit is used to prevent a temperature drop and the potentially harmful aftereffects of hypothermia (sluggishness, abnormal blood sugar levels, lung problems, and others) or to warm a baby who has become chilled.

Disadvantages of the warming unit: The baby is separated from the parents. Also, warming units are not risk-free; they may cause the baby to lose fluids through evaporation of moisture from the skin and lungs (breathing out moist air). This is a greater potential problem for premature babies, but fluid loss and signs of dehydration must be monitored carefully. Breast-feeding often, feeding water or formula, or giving IV fluids to the baby and adjusting the heat in the warming unit are the most common solutions, but being held skin to skin with the birthing person is the best solution (see page 135).

Alternatives to consider: Prevent chills in the baby by drying with towels right after the birth and protecting the baby from cool air. The baby should be kept warm by staying skin to skin with the birthing parent (see "Kangaroo Care," page 135 and Recommended Resources, page 190), putting on a hat, and covering the birthing person and baby with a warm blanket. The baby's temperature should be checked frequently with a quick-action thermometer. If it is not possible to do these things because the baby needs medical attention, the warming unit becomes a necessity. If the birthing person is not ready to hold the baby, you might hold the baby skin to skin with a blanket around the two of you.

FIRST FEEDING

The following applies to those who plan to breastfeed or chest-feed. During all this clean-up activity, the birthing parent should lie back in a propped position, with pillows beneath both arms, and hold the baby on their chest so they can nurse as soon as they are ready. This is called the laid-back breastfeeding position (developed by Suzanne Colson; see Recommended Resources, page 190). If not rushed, the newborn is fully able to self-at-tach, that is, find their way to the breast. In their own time, they'll nuzzle, mouth the breast, salivate, and bob their head until they open their mouth wide and place it right on the nipple. Then, they begin to suckle. The nurse, doula, or midwife can help the baby "latch on" (form the connection between mouth and breast tissue) to the breast by leaving the birthing parent and baby together for up to an hour while resisting the urge to take the breast in one hand and direct the baby's mouth onto it with the other hand. Modeling patience and reassurance and not rushing the process is the best way to help the breastfeeding pair get started.

If staff are in a hurry to get the baby nursing or if the birthing parent becomes upset, ask the nurse or doula for help to gently encourage the baby to take the nipple.

If you plan to formula-feed your baby, watch for the same cues they show that they are ready for breastfeeding. When the baby is ready for latching on to the breast is the right time to feed them from the bottle.

THE FIRST FEW DAYS FOR THE BABY

Once both birthing parent and baby are settled, the three of you can relax together, cooing, cuddling, exploring, and nursing—or simply sleeping. There is usually no reason to be separated after birth, although for a long time it was (and still is in some places) a hospital custom to do so. If the birthing parent or baby is not well, the baby may have to go to the nursery or may stay in the room but the birthing parent may be unable to hold the baby.

You are the perfect person to hold the baby if the birthing parent cannot (and even if they can) or to remain with the baby in the nursery, as long as both you and the birthing parent wish for you to do so. If you cuddle with the baby sometime during the first day or so after birth, you will have even stronger feelings for your child. There is something magical about holding your baby close—especially skin to skin—gazing at each other and talking or singing to your beautiful child. We overheard one father saying to his baby as he held him close, "And when you're six, we'll take you horseback riding in Montana!" The baby seemed to approve. They were planning their lives together.

Physical Exam and Assessment

A doctor or a midwife will give the baby a thorough physical exam, checking the entire body and all systems. It is interesting to watch the exam, which can teach you a great deal about the baby. Over the next few days, you, the birthing parent, or staff will make these observations of the baby: the number and quality of both wet diapers and bowel movements; frequency and length of time in feeding; respiration rate; temperature; pulse; and so forth. The staff will teach you how to do these assessments because they will be your responsibility for the first few days at home with the baby.

Bowel Movements

The baby will have a bowel movement within a few hours after birth. This and the next several bowel movements are composed of meconium, and they are different from bowel movements that will come later. Meconium is thick, black, sticky, and hard to clean. If you think of it, soon after birth, rub some vegetable oil or massage oil all over the baby's buttocks and genitals. This will make cleaning off the meconium easier, and you will thank us.

Over the next few days, as the birthing person's milk shifts from colostrum (see page 166) to mature milk, the baby's bowel movements will change from black to brown to green to yellow and will become very runny and almost odorless or slightly sweet-smelling. After the first few days, the baby may have a bowel movement after almost every feeding and should have at least four per day. This is a good sign they are getting enough to eat.

Bathing the Baby

The baby will have a bath within the first couple of days. As we have gained knowledge of the baby's microbiome, it has become clear that the substances on the baby's skin at

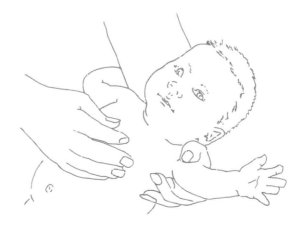

The safe way to hold a baby during a bath

birth—vernix, amniotic fluid, including the vaginal secretions the baby picked up coming through the birth canal—contain microbes that provide protection for the baby against some potentially harmful bacteria, such as Group B streptococcus, *E. coli*, and others. The vernix also protects and moisturizes the baby's skin. Many people now wait 24 hours or more before giving the first bath.

Caring for the Cord

Before being cut, the umbilical cord is either tied tightly with umbilical cord tape or clamped with a plastic clip. The cord stump needs to be kept clean and dry. Arrange the baby's diaper so it does not touch the cord. Clean the cord with tap or bottled water. The nurse or midwife will show you how. The cord clamp is removed by the nurse or midwife, usually on the second day, leaving a black, dry stump that remains for a week or two and then drops off. The cord usually has a faintly foul smell, but call the baby's doctor if pus or red blood oozes from it.

Feeding the Baby

For the first six months, breastfed babies need no food but colostrum (the first "milk" to come from the breasts) and breast milk, which increases in volume at 3 to 5 days of age (often referred to as your milk "coming in"). They do not need formula or water, and they do not need glucose water unless they have low blood sugar that is not corrected by breast-feeding. It is a good idea to begin breastfeeding as soon after birth as the baby is interested, usually within 20 to 60 minutes (see page 164).

Babies who will be formula-fed should begin receiving formula when they seem ready to suck and when their condition is stable.

Newborn Screening Tests

Every state and province has a newborn screening program. Through the heel-stick test, these programs can detect numerous rare endocrinological, metabolic, and hematologic disorders, most of which, if detected early, can be treated to prevent mental, developmental, and other serious disabilities or early death. As of this writing, the March of Dimes recommends screening for at least 34 specific congenital health problems, and 30 states do that, while other states screen for fewer disorders. One heel stick can usually provide enough blood for the tiny samples needed for all these tests.

HEARING SCREENING TEST

Approximately 2 to 4 babies per 1,000 are born deaf or hard of hearing. Within the first few days, your baby will probably be given a hearing test to identify any hearing problem much earlier than you and the birthing person would notice them (the average age at which hearing problems are identified without the screening test is 14 months, by which time the child already has fallen behind in speech development). Identifying hearing problems early allows for early therapy.

The test is done while the baby is asleep. The baby wears headphones, and several electrodes are placed around their head. They record brain-wave activity and middle-ear activity in response to sounds transmitted into the baby's ears and via the bones of their head.

If the test indicates a problem or the results are unclear, there is more testing. If repeat tests indicate the baby has impaired hearing, you will be referred to a hearing specialist and speech therapist. Early detection and treatment of hearing loss has greatly improved the hearing and communication skills of affected children.

Circumcision

The decision whether to circumcise a baby's penis is a highly personal one. Most major medical groups, including the American Academy of Pediatrics (AAP) and the Canadian Paediatric Society, advise that parents learn about the pros and cons, explore their own values, and decide as they see fit. The following section outlines the health benefits listed in the AAP statement. The statement calls for health insurance companies to cover circumcision. (See Recommended Resources, page 190 for a link to the 2012 statement and other information on circumcision.)

If the baby will be circumcised, the procedure is done in the hospital on the first or second day after birth or, in the Jewish tradition, in the home or synagogue on the eighth day. When circumcision is done in the hospital, and sometimes as part of the Jewish bris ceremony, the penis is usually numbed with local anesthetic. The foreskin is separated from the underlying glans (the end of the penis) and removed from the glans with a scalpel.

The incidence of circumcision in the United States is now estimated at about 55 percent, with regional variation—lowest in the western United States and highest in the Midwest. Rates are lower in states where the procedure is not covered by Medicaid insurance. In Canada, the rate is considerably lower, about 20 percent.

Purposes and benefits of circumcision:

- The surgery changes the appearance of the penis according to the parents' preferences.
- The surgery is done to observe Jewish or other religious customs.
- The surgery reduces the child's later chances of acquiring some sexually transmitted diseases (STDs) from an infected person. Studies in developing nations in Africa indicate that circumcised heterosexual men have a lower incidence of many kinds of STDs, including HIV/AIDS. There is controversy over the applicability of these studies to the culture of North America.
- The surgery reduces the risk of cancer of the penis in later life. Although this cancer is very rare, affecting only 1 to 2 males in 100,000, it is almost nonexistent in circumcised males. Long-term poor hygiene and old age are the other factors associated with penile cancer. The American Cancer Society does not recommend newborn circumcision to prevent cancer of the penis.

Urinary tract infections in the first year of life are rare, but more frequent in uncircumcised babies. It may be that instruction in proper care and hygiene for the uncircumcised penis would lower that risk.

Other health-related reasons for circumcision have been less well studied, and their validity hasn't been established. For more information about these, see Recommended Resources, page 190.

Disadvantages of circumcision: Circumcision carries the same risks as all surgery—infection, hemorrhage, adhesions, pain, and injury due to human error.

- The procedure is very painful unless anesthesia is used. A local anesthetic is usually injected in several places at the base of the penis to reduce the pain. Although the injections are painful, they prevent pain during the circumcision itself. Sometimes, instead of being injected, anesthetic cream is applied to the penis, but a wait of 20 minutes is needed for the cream to take effect, so it is not widely used in hospitals.
- Infection or hemorrhage occurs in about 1 in every 200 circumcisions. These conditions can usually be well controlled with medications and extra time in the hospital.
- There is a small possibility, especially with an inexperienced, unsupervised doctor, that the surgery will be done poorly—too much or too little foreskin may be removed.
- The circumcised penis usually takes 7 to 10 days to heal. Parents are taught how to care for the penis during this time by avoiding wet diapers and other irritations, applying a lubricating ointment to the penis, and observing the penis for signs of poor healing.
- If the newborn child is ill or if their penis is abnormal in structure, circumcision may be harmful.

Alternatives to consider. The baby's parents can:

- Leave the baby uncircumcised. If you do, learn proper care of the uncircumcised penis (see Recommended Resources, page 190). Do not forcefully retract your baby's foreskin to clean it or for any other reason. At birth, most of the foreskin adheres to the glans of the penis. Over a period of months or years, it gradually loosens and becomes easily retractable. Many of the problems attributed to being uncircumcised are really caused by parents and others who do not know to leave the foreskin alone. As your child grows, teach them proper hygiene; washing the penis is about as complicated as washing the ears.
- Decide to have the baby circumcised, with appropriate anesthesia and an experienced doctor or mohel (a Jewish person with training in circumcision). If possible, remain with the baby to comfort them. Learn proper care for the newly circumcised penis to promote healing.
- Leave the decision for the child to make himself when they reach adulthood.

Whether you choose to circumcise your baby or not, you will later want to teach them responsible sexual practices to protect themselves and their partners from sexually transmitted infections.

Baby Care

The nurse or midwife and friends and family who are experienced parents can teach you many baby care skills not covered in this book, such as safety measures, changing diapers, bathing, and soothing a fussy baby. Books, videos, and classes are also available; see Recommended Resources, page 190.

THE FIRST FEW DAYS FOR THE BIRTHING PARENT

For the birthing parent, the early postpartum period is marked by fatigue, emotional highs and lows, preoccupation with the baby, curiosity, some pain, and an array of physical changes that affect most parts of the body.

They may be tired and excited at the same time, finding it difficult to sleep, but unable to do very much without feeling worn out. A shower or a short walk is enough to send them straight back to bed.

They may be surprised by the variety of physical changes they experience; these physical changes will require more attention than they ever expected.

Afterpains

These are uterine contractions that come and go. Especially if this is the second child or more, the birthing parent's afterpains may be quite intense when suckling the baby. Afterpains are a good sign that the uterus is returning to its pre-pregnant size. Remind them to use relaxation and breathing techniques. If the pains are severe, they can request pain medications. Afterpains go away in a few days.

Vaginal Discharge

The birthing parent will have a bloody vaginal discharge, called lochia, which is similar to a menstrual period. It starts as a heavy red flow containing some clots and gradually diminishes; it lasts from two to six weeks.

In the first few days after the birth, the birthing parent may notice they pass very little blood while lying down, but when they stand up after a few hours in bed, they may suddenly lose a lot of blood. This can be alarming, but it is probably because blood may pool in the vagina until gravity causes it to flow out. If heavy bleeding continues longer than a few minutes, however, or if the birthing parent feels faint, call the caregiver or the hospital's maternity floor.

After the lochia has clearly subsided but then suddenly increases or if the birthing parent passes large, golf ball–size clots, call the caregiver because they may be bleeding from a blood vessel in the former site of the placenta. Sometimes, heavy physical exertion causes one to bleed heavily after the lochia has decreased. Rest usually puts an end to the heavy bleeding, but you should call the birthing parent's caregiver if you are concerned.

The Perineum

After a vaginal birth, the perineum will be sore, especially if stitches were needed. Even with no stitches, there may be swelling and bruising. The birthing person can try the following comfort measures:

- Apply an ice pack, especially during the first 24 hours. Damp washcloths, folded and placed in a plastic bag in the freezer for 1 hour or so, make great ice packs. Make up several at a time, so you'll always have one available.
- Sit in a bath of warm water for 20 minutes, two or three times a day. They should not wash in this water; it should be kept clean.

- After using the toilet, carefully pat the perineum dry (starting at the front and moving toward the anus) or squirt it with warm water from a bottle. This is less irritating than wiping with toilet paper.
- Apply witch hazel–soaked pads to the perineum and to hemorrhoids for soothing. For other hemorrhoid treatments, consult the caregiver.
- Do the 10-second pelvic-floor contraction exercise (Kegel exercise) ten times per day to promote healing, reduce swelling, and restore strength. They should always do these while sitting, which helps keep the buttocks from spreading and putting painful stress on the stitches. The birthing parent tightens the muscles around the vagina and urethra as when trying to hold back urine (see page 10). They should do ten per day, probably not all at once. Also, they should follow the directions on page 10 to restore pelvic floor muscle tone. The good news is, improvement can be detected rapidly when exercising these muscles.

Emptying Bowels and Bladder

You may be surprised how preoccupied the birthing parent becomes with bowel movements and urination! These functions are more difficult than usual because the perineum is sore, abdominal muscles are temporarily weak (making straining to move the bowels difficult), and the interruption in food and fluid intake during labor may have caused constipation.

If unable to urinate, try all the tricks—run a faucet, have them urinate in the bath (and get out when done) or shower, and encourage them to press in on their low abdomen just above the pubic bone, putting pressure on the bladder—but not if they had a cesarean!—which may encourage emptying. These almost always work; in the unlikely event that the birthing person does not urinate within a half day or so, call the caregiver. They may need to have a catheter placed in the bladder to empty it. This is unpleasant, but it is better than letting the bladder become distended.

On a positive note, one very welcome change is that the bladder, no longer crowded by the baby, has much greater capacity than during pregnancy, so the birthing parent will need to urinate less frequently.

To help the birthing parent avoid or reduce difficulties with the first bowel movements after giving birth, remind them to eat and drink high- fiber foods: prune juice, other juices, raw fruits and vegetables, bran breads or cereals, and so forth. Bulk-producing stool softeners or laxatives are also helpful. In addition, it might reduce discomfort if they support their sore perineum by pressing toilet paper against it as they have a bowel movement. These measures also help if a person has painful hemorrhoids.

It may take a week or two for the birthing parent to resume their usual bowel patterns. If they're feel uncomfortable or constipated despite the measures described, they should contact the caregiver.

Pain Following Cesarean Delivery

Post-cesarean pain results from the incision, from the stitches or clamps closing it, and from gas that commonly builds up in the abdomen after this surgery. Activities such as turning over, getting out of bed, walking, and nursing the baby are usually very painful for a few days, even though some activity of that kind hastens recovery. Help as much as you can to make these activities easier for the birthing parent by reminding them of how to roll from back to side, giving a helping hand as they get out of bed, offering a supportive arm as they walk, and providing a pillow for their lap as they nurse the baby. The birthing parent will begin feeling better gradually each day.

Clamps are removed from the incision site on the second or third day after the delivery. The procedure is not very painful, and the pain from the incision will then decrease. If the birthing parent had stitches, they may dissolve over time or be removed within the first week, depending on the material used for suturing. The birthing parent may feel itching and soreness at the incision site and should not use any soothing cream except what the doctor suggests.

Keep an eye on the scar as it heals. If it becomes inflamed or produces pus or a fever develops, call the caregiver.

To help reduce abdominal pain, encourage the birthing parent to do the following:

- When rolling from back to side, they first bend the knees so their feet are flat on the bed. Then, lift their hips (so only their head, shoulders, and feet are on the bed), twist them to one side, and roll their shoulders to the side (see illustration below). This is much easier and far less painful than rolling over the usual way.

   To sit up from the side-lying position, they should push themselves up with their hands. These techniques avoid strain on the incision.

- The birthing parent should avoid gas-producing foods such as lentils and beans, foods in the cabbage family, and cold or carbonated beverages.

- To avoid feeling faint when getting of bed the first few times, the birthing parent should first circle their ankles, raise their arms above their head several times, and then sit up and raise their arms several more times. As they stand, you should stand close by so they can hold on to you.

- When holding the baby on their lap, they should place a pillow over the incision to protect it.

   The birthing parent should ask the nurse or lactation consultant to show ways to hold the baby to avoid pressure on the incision.

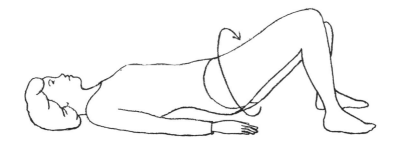

To reduce pain when rolling from back to side, the birthing person who has had a cesarean should raise the hips and rotate the hips and legs to the side before turning the shoulders.

GETTING HELP AND ADVICE

Check the birthing parent's insurance plan ahead of time to learn what to expect and what options they have after the birth. The usual hospital stay after a normal vaginal birth is 24 to 48 hours; after a cesarean, it is 48 to 72 hours. If the birth takes place in a birth center, the birthing parent will likely go home 3 to 6 hours afterward. After a home birth, the midwife usually stays.

When you arrive home, you both may feel like celebrating—and with good reason! You're introducing the baby to their new world. The birthing parent may feel they have has been away a long time (even though it has probably been only a few days!) and may be relieved to be in familiar surroundings. Fatigue is likely to set in very soon. Perhaps the best thing for the birthing parent to do is get right into bed, snuggle with their loved ones, and bask in the warm feelings. Consider asking visitors not to come until at least the next day.

The two of you will have your hands full, maintaining the household, feeding your-selves, and getting to know and care for the new baby, especially as all these tasks must be carried out in the midst of disrupted sleep schedules and the birthing parent's post-partum adjustments. The brightest spot in all this is your baby. The baby certainly makes it all worthwhile, but is there anything that could also make it a bit easier? The answer is yes—help!

Accept any and all offers of help from family and friends. Errand running, meal prepa-ration, phone calls, housework—all can be done by someone else. The best kind of help, however, is availability whenever you need it—day or night. Getting such help may not be possible unless you are fortunate enough to have a relative or close friend who can fit comfortably into the chaos. If you are very lucky, grandparents or other helpful relatives or friends will come every day to help as needed. Or maybe, the baby's grandmother or aunt can come to stay for a week or two. She can keep the household running smoothly, feed you both, and answer questions about baby care. You will want to make sure this person can foster the postpartum parent's self-confidence in meeting the baby's needs. This is no time for parental strife to rear its ugly head..

One way to ensure harmony is to invite the person most preferred by the birthing per-son and to plan the visit for when the two of you prefer it—perhaps immediately after the birth or perhaps one or two weeks later. It also makes sense to specify what you think you need from this person: "We are going to need help running the household and cooking because Jane gets really upset when the place gets messy." Or, "We've never been around babies. We need someone who can show us what to do, what's normal, how to take care of our baby."

Postpartum doulas are a great solution to the problem of new family adjustment. These trained helpers can be hired for blocks of several hours every day or every other day for a period of a week or many weeks. Some offer overnight support. It's like having your favorite aunt (who had lots of kids!) helping with whatever you need; see Recom-mended Resources (page 190) to locate one.

For more discussion of ways to smooth the adjustment to becoming parents, see chapter 1.

POSTPARTUM EMOTIONS

During the early postpartum period, the birthing parent's emotions are changeable and unpredictable. One moment, they may be rapturous and full of energy; the next, tired, frustrated, and in tears. The sudden changes in hormone production and body functions—as they go from supporting the growth of a fetus during pregnancy to expelling the baby to producing milk while returning to a nonpregnant state—take an emotional toll. Add to this the inevitable fatigue from loss of sleep during labor and for weeks after the birth, as well as the stress of a profound role change, and it is not surprising there are emotional ups and downs.

If you are the birthing parent's spouse or life partner as well as birth partner, you have your own share of emotional adjustments—the role change to parenthood, your own fatigue, and a complete disruption in lifestyle. Even if you are a relative or a friend who is helping out temporarily, you are probably tired from the birth experience and from the strain of caring for the birthing parent and the new baby.

As two tired people with a great many needs, you will be sustained through this stressful time by your underlying feelings for each other and by the joy and commitment you share in having your new baby. It helps to know this situation *will* get better. Following are suggestions for getting through the emotional ups and downs of the first few days after the baby is born.

Baby Blues

You may be caught off guard if the birthing parent seems sad or cries a lot or has mood swings from depressed to very happy or irritable, without an apparent reason. You may feel helpless or guilty, believing you are to blame or that it is up to you to make things right. You may worry about the birthing parent; you may feel angry or wonder whether this situation is permanent.

When a new postpartum parent experiences these kinds of emotional ups and downs in the first week or two after the birth, we first think of the "baby blues," a common state in the early postpartum period, with all its physical, emotional and hormonal changes, new responsibilities, lack of sleep, and a mysterious totally dependent little person to feed and care for. What can you do to help? Here are some suggestions:

- First of all, ask what you can do to help. The birthing parent may or may not have an answer. They may not know why they are crying. It may simply be a need to cry without you and other people feeling you must help them get over it. Accept their need to cry with patience, tenderness, and empathy. They might appreciate a warm hug while the tears flow.
- Do not blame yourself if you did nothing to cause the crying.
- Know that almost every birthing parent sheds tears and goes on an emotional roller coaster for a few days after childbirth. Emotions are close to the surface at this time, likely because of the abrupt changes in hormone production that take place with birth.

- Realize this will likely not last more than a few days. Be patient.
- Encourage naps and rest (see "Recipe for Getting Enough Sleep," page 176). Lack of sleep can interfere with anyone's mood and confidence.
- Ask friends and relatives, especially those who have given birth, to visit, if the birthing parent seems to feel isolated or lonely.
- Call the caregiver, childbirth educator, or lactation consultant if you are worried.
- Enlist the assistance of a postpartum doula or someone else who understands and can help the birthing parent and give you perspective.
- Investigate new parent groups or postpartum classes. They are becoming very popular as settings where people get support from others and can share and discuss feelings and practical tips.

Sometimes, blue feelings continue without letup for more than a week. If this is happening or if you feel under undue pressure, the birthing parent may have postpartum depression, anxiety, or another mood disorder. Discuss your concerns with them and call the resource people already mentioned.

Ask the birthing parent to go over "Unhappiness After Childbirth: A Self-Assessment" (see below) with you, as a way to clarify their feelings. This self-assessment is an adaptation of a very widely used questionnaire to help a health care professional diagnose a postpartum mood disorder. We include it here to help the birthing parent think about their current feelings and help them recognize that they are not "themselves" and that they deserve some support in overcoming the unhappiness they are feeling. A referral from their caregiver to a social worker, psychologist, or psychiatrist for counseling or therapy may be appropriate and very helpful. A complete physical exam, with blood tests to check levels of various hormones, including thyroid tests, might reveal a physical condition contributing to depression. Or, a support group alone might help the person recover from the depression. Consider these options if the birthing parent is unhappy most of the time. See Recommended Resources (page 190) for online support.

UNHAPPINESS AFTER CHILDBIRTH: A SELF-ASSESSMENT

1. I have been able to laugh and see the funny side of things...
a. as much as I always could
b. not quite as much as I used to
c. definitely not as much as I used to

2. I have looked forward with enjoyment to things...
a. as much as I always could
b. not quite as much as I used to
c. definitely not as much as I used to
d. not at all

3. I have blamed myself unnecessarily when things went wrong...
a. not at all
b. very little
c. some of the time
d. most of the time

4. I have been anxious or worried for no good reason...
a. not at all
b. very little
c. some of the time
d. most of the time

5. I have felt scared or panicked for no good reason...

a. not at all
b. very little
c. some of the time
d. most of the time

6. I have been feeling overwhelmed...

a. not at all; I've been coping very well.
b. very little; I've been coping pretty well.
c. some of the time; I haven't been coping as well as usual
d. quite a lot; I haven't been able to cope at all.

7. I have been so unhappy that I've had difficulty sleeping, even when the baby is asleep and the house is quiet...

a. not at all
b. very little
c. some of the time
d. most of the time

8. I have felt sad or miserable...

a. not at all
b. very little
c. some of the time
d. most of the time

9. I have been so unhappy I've been crying

a. not at all
b. very little
c. some of the time
d. most of the time

10. The thought of harming myself or my baby has occurred to me...

a. not at all
b. very little
c. some of the time
d. most of the time

After reviewing this form, if you have feel something isn't right or if you have any questions about your emotional well-being, please contact your caregiver, childbirth educator, doula, or a mental health therapist. Or contact Postpartum Support International (www.postpartum.net or 1-800-944-4773).

Adapted from Cox, J. L., Holden, J. M., and Sagovsky, R. 1987. Detection of Postnatal Depression: Development of the 10-Item Edinburgh Postnatal Depression Scale. *British Journal of Psychiatry* 150:782–86.

WHAT ABOUT YOUR FEELINGS?

Becoming a parent has its thrills and joys, but if you are the baby's parent and/or the birthing parent's life partner, you are also making huge emotional adjustments and lifestyle changes in a state of fatigue and constant demands. Many partners find this rather chaotic and unpredictable time exciting and satisfying, but others feel depressed or stressed at times. Even though your needs seem to rank low in the hierarchy, you deserve time for yourself—to sleep, see your friends, and get a break. Why don't you and the postpartum parent plan for you to take a few hours' break when someone else is there? Make a date with yourself and do something you like to do. You'll be refreshed and glad to reconnect with your family!

Sometimes, the partner's feelings are more than just needing some time to relax and refresh. Approximately 10 percent of fathers have been found to experience postpartum depression. Other co-parents may have similar challenges. You might benefit from going over the Unhappiness After Childbirth Questionnaire (page 174) and seeking help if you feel you're suffering more than you realized.

PRACTICAL MATTERS AT HOME

Much of the turmoil of the postpartum period can be avoided if you're prepared for it in advance and if you can simplify your lives for a while. The following suggestions will help all of you get through these first days until the household becomes more settled.

Fatigue and Sleep Deprivation

The birthing parent is tired. You are probably tired, too. If after being the birth partner you are now the "at home" support person, you are probably running out of energy. Sleep deprivation is a serious problem among new parents that is often ignored. In the lactating parent, it may cause inadequate milk supply; severe mood swings (including postpartum mood disorders); and the inability to deal calmly with the baby's crying, other minor annoyances, and even simple decisions (what to have for dinner, for instance). Fatigue makes *everything* worse, and adequate rest makes *everything* better—the lactating parent's appetite, feelings toward the baby and toward you, their mood, their milk supply, their patience, and so on.

Many people simply resign themselves to the belief that all new parents, especially birthing parents, cannot possibly get enough sleep. This is not true. It is possible, but to do so you and the birthing parent must give sleep a very high priority (right after making sure the baby is fed, clean, and cared for) and restructure your lives to ensure you both get enough. It does not work for the birthing parent to simply "sleep when the baby sleeps," as most are advised to do.

Until things settle into a comfortable routine, give a high priority to getting enough sleep. Unplug the phone and keep a DO NOT DISTURB sign on the front door until one of you is ready to get up. For the first several weeks after the birth, try very hard not to schedule any appointments before noon—any earlier is too early!

The "Recipe for Getting Enough Sleep" (see following) is very effective for ensuring sufficient sleep for both parents. It is based on the requirement that neither of you gets out of bed in the morning until you have had the amount of sleep you need to function well. This is most helpful if the baby is the only child in your family.

RECIPE FOR GETTING ENOUGH SLEEP

This advice applies to both parents until the breadwinner(s) returns to employment. Then, that person will have to get more sleep at night and less during the day. Start this technique the first night you are home.

Ask yourselves how many hours of sleep you each need every 24 hours to function well. Six hours? Eight hours? Nine? That is the amount of sleep you owe yourselves every day. The recipe spells out how to get that amount of sleep.

As you cannot get this amount of sleep in one stretch, due to interruptions for feedings and baby care, you will require more hours in bed to get your allotted amount of sleep. It is likely that if you spend 8 hours in bed as a new parent, you may sleep only 4 or 5 hours of that time.

Keep a mental note of approximately how much time you have slept at each stretch and stay in bed in your nightclothes until you have slept the required number of hours. Plan to stay in bed or keep going back to bed until you have slept your allotted number of hours. It might take 12 hours or more! This means that, except for meals and trips to the bathroom, you do not get up in the early morning.

Then, brush your teeth, take a shower, get dressed, and greet the day! You might even want to stay in bed all day for the first few days after birth. The good news is, over time, the nursing parent and baby become more efficient at nursing and sleep for longer intervals, so it takes less time to get the necessary amount of sleep.

Many parents find it easier to follow this advice if the baby sleeps with them or nearby.

At first glance, it may seem impossible to follow this recipe. It does require putting a very high priority on sleep. Keep in mind that fatigue or sleep deprivation contributes to reduction in milk supply, mood swings, anxiety, strained relationships, and less joy in parenting.

PLATOON SLEEPING

This arrangement may be the best way to increase sleep for both of you. It works this way: Right after the baby is fed in the early evening, one parent is in charge of the baby (awake or asleep) and any older children while the other parent sleeps in the evening; then, the parent who sleeps in the evening gets up early in the morning, so the other can sleep in the morning.

When it is your turn to stay up, rock and talk and bounce and walk and soothe the baby as long as they are awake. If the baby is asleep, you can doze, watch TV, or get something done. Try to give the early-to-bed parent 2 to 3 hours of sleep, but when the baby really wants to eat, take the baby to the lactating or feeding parent. Then, you both sleep, or try to, with intermittent feedings and diaper changes. You carry on in this way until the early-to-bed parent has had the amount of sleep required. They then get up with the baby, allowing you a few extra hours of sleep.

With platoon sleeping—theoretically, at least—you each get a stretch of unbroken sleep, plus several hours of intermittent sleep.

Fussy, Crying Baby

Entire books have been written about fussy babies, and comprehensive baby care books contain sections on the topic (see Recommended Resources, page 190).

To learn a successful step-by-step approach to soothing a crying baby, see Recommended Resources, page 190.

Don't leave a tiny baby crying. The first few days after birth are a time of major adjustment for the baby, as they are for the birthing parent and for you. A newborn needs the comfort and security of feeling your warm bodies and hearing your voices close by. Do not worry about spoiling the baby: You cannot spoil someone by meeting their basic needs.

Scheduling the Baby's Sleeping and Feeding

Don't even try to get the baby on a schedule in the first few weeks. Instead, discover the baby's own schedule and pattern your life around that. Focus on meeting the baby's needs; figure out how they tell you they are hungry, curious, interested, bored, uncomfortable, or overstimulated. Let the baby call the shots. It is much easier for the household to adjust to the baby at first than to make the baby adjust to the household. Make it your goal to meet the baby's needs, as they express them—you will all be happier if you do. Read *Your Amazing Newborn* and *Your Baby Is Speaking to You* (see Recommended Resources, page 190) to help you understand the baby.

Meals

Time for meal preparation hardly exists during the busy first days at home, yet good food, quickly available, is a must. Try the following:

- Prepare meals in advance. Before the birth, prepare a few dishes—such as soups, casseroles, and stews—that will either keep for several days or can be frozen.
- Purchase quick, nutritious, tasty foods. Foods that need little or no preparation—that you can grab and eat—are good choices for the first few weeks. Such foods include yogurt, fruit, granola and nuts, cottage cheese, hard cheeses, raw vegetables, cold cuts, and whole-grain breads and crackers. Plan to have these on hand before the birth so you won't have to go shopping right away. This is the time, too, to search the deli counter and frozen food section at the grocery store for nourishing, delicious prepared food. You may be able to order groceries or meals delivered to you
- Prepare foods that last for a while. For example, you can roast a turkey and pick from it for a week or wash, cut, and chill raw vegetables to keep in the refrigerator for munching.
- Accept food from friends and relatives. If people ask how they can help, tell them you'd love a main dish. Sometimes, a group of friends establishes a "meal train" in which each signs up to provide one or more meals over the course of a week or two. Visit Mealtrain.com to prepare an online sign-up schedule. One hint: Ask your friends to bring food only every other day. People usually bring more than one meal's worth, so you can find your refrigerator overflowing after a few days of daily contributions. Besides, if you ask for meals only every other day, your friends may keep the meal train going for a longer period, or they may be willing to offer services other than food, such as walking the dog, running errands, doing laundry, etc.
- Remember the birth parent's dietary needs. The postpartum diet should be as good as the pregnancy diet. If breastfeeding, they will need 200 to 300 calories more than normal each day. They will also need at least 2 quarts (1.9 L) of liquids each day.

Household Chores

The first few days at home are busy and full of adjustments. Do yourselves a big favor: If you have no help, plan to do the minimum in the way of household chores—just enough to maintain sanity. It may be easier if you have "supercleaned" before the baby was born; if you haven't, just close your eyes and let things accumulate for a while. Simplify your lives so you are free to care for and enjoy the baby and to get enough rest.

If you do have help, do not be shy about asking for what you really want done. One advantage of a postpartum doula is they are there to do what you need done, not to enjoy the new baby (though they will!) and your company, and you don't need to worry about offending them. They won't even mind wearing the baby in a sling while doing some chores or preparing a meal, allowing the two of you a chance for a nap!

In conclusion, the first days and weeks postpartum are a time of adjustment: for the birthing parent as their body returns to a nonpregnant state and begins making milk and feeding the baby; for you both, as you get to know your baby, develop baby care skills, adjust to the changes in sleep, learn your parenting roles, take on a new lifestyle, and explore your relationship with each other; and for your baby, who must learn about their new world, their parents, and the sights and sounds outside the womb. You will never be the same—nor will you want to be.

LABOR AND BIRTH PLANNERS

Photography and video:

Photos encouraged (+ video)

Culturally significant rituals and practices:

CONTINGENCY PLANS FOR THE UNEXPECTED:

PACKING LIST FOR THE HOSPITAL OR BIRTH CENTER

FOR THE MOTHER DURING LABOR

_____   _____
_____   _____
_____   _____
_____   _____
_____   _____
_____   _____
_____   _____
_____   _____

FOR THE BIRTH PARTNER

_____   _____
_____   _____
_____   _____
_____   _____
_____   _____
_____   _____
_____   _____

SUPPLIES FOR THE POSTPARTUM PERIOD

_____   _____
_____   _____
_____   _____

FOR THE BABY

_____   _____
_____   _____
_____   _____
_____   _____

SUPPLIES LIST FOR A HOME BIRTH

BIRTHING SUPPLIES

FOR THE MOTHER DURING LABOR

FOR THE BIRTH PARTNER

SUPPLIES FOR THE POSTPARTUM PERIOD

FOR THE BABY

COUNTING FETAL MOVEMENTS

DATE	STARTING TIME	MOVEMENTS	TIME OF TENTH MOVEMENT	TIME ELAPSED

EARLY LABOR RECORD

Date _____

TIME CONTRACTION STARTS	DURATION (Seconds)	INTERVAL (Minutes from Start of One to Start of Next)	COMMENTS (Contraction Strength, Foods Eaten, Coping Method, Vaginal Discharge, etc.)

Recommended Resources

The following are books, video recordings, and websites that provide helpful information to supplement this book.

To contact Penny Simkin:
www.pennysimkin.com;
info@pennysimkin.com

Penny Simkin's Social Media:
YouTube Channel: www.youtube.com/psfrompenny Facebook: www.facebook.com/PennySimkinChildbirth Instagram: @penny.simkin

To contact Katie Rohs: www.birthtastic.com; katie@birthtastic.com

AIDS FOR RELAXATION

Schardt, Dana. 2000. *Pregnancy Relaxation: A Guide to Peaceful Beginnings*. CD.

Simkin, Penny. 2008. *Comfort Measures for Childbirth*. DVD. www.pennysimkin.com.

Simkin, Penny, Bettina Paek. 2019. An App for Comfort and Progress in Labor. www.pennysimkin.com

Simkin, Penny. *Relaxation, Rhythm, Ritual: The 3 Rs of Childbirth*. Downloadable video. www.pennysimkin.com/shop.

AROMATHERAPY

Aromatherapy for Childbirth: www.aromatherapyforchildbirth.org.

Clark, Demetria. 2015. *Aromatherapy and Herbal Remedies for Pregnancy, Birth, and Breastfeeding*.

BABY CARE, SUPPLIES, AND INFANT SLEEP

American Academy of Pediatrics website for parents: www.kidshealth.org.

BabyCenter: Clothing, supplies, equipment for baby www.babycenter.com/baby-products-and-gear.

Klaus, Marshall H., and Phyllis H. Klaus. 2000. *The Amazing Talents of the Newborn*. DVD. www.pennysimkin.com.

Klaus, Marshall H., and Phyllis H. Klaus. 2000. *Your Amazing Newborn*.

Leach, Penelope. 2010. *Your Baby & Child: From Birth to Age Five*.

McKenna, James J. 2007. *Sleeping with Your Baby: A Parent's Guide to Cosleeping*.

Nugent, Kevin. 2011. *Your Baby Is Speaking to You: A Visual Guide to the Amazing Behaviors of Your Newborn and Growing Baby*.

Pantley, Elizabeth. 2003. *Gentle Baby Care: No-Cry, No-Fuss, No-Worry—Essential Tips for Raising Your Baby*.

Sears, William, Martha Sears, Robert Sears, and James Sears. 2013. *The Baby Book: Everything You Need to Know About Your Baby from Birth to Age Two*, revised ed.

BED REST SUPPORT

Sidelines: www.sidelines.org.

BREASTFEEDING/CHEST-FEEDING

Birth International. *Biological Nurturing—Laid-Back Breastfeeding*. DVD. www.birthinternational.com/product/biological-nurturing-dvd.

Breastfeeding USA: www.breastfeedingusa.org.

Find a lactation consultant: www.uslca.org/resources/find-a-lactation-consultant-map#!directory/map.

Getting Started with Breastfeeding from Stanford Medicine has lots of outstanding videos about early breastfeeding: med.stanford.edu/newborns/professional-education/breastfeeding.html.

Huggins, Kathleen. 2017. *The Nursing Mother's Companion*, 7th ed.

KellyMom: www.kellymom.com.

La Leche League International: www.llli.org.

Mohrbacher, Nancy, and Kathleen Kendall-Tackett. 2010. *Breastfeeding Made Simple: Seven Natural Laws for Nursing Mothers*, 2nd ed.

Newman, Jack. *Dr. Jack Newman's Visual Guide to Breastfeeding*. DVD. www. breastfeedinginc.ca.

Newman, Jack, and Teresa Pitman. 2006. *The Ultimate Breastfeeding Book of Answers*, revised ed.

Special Supplemental Nutrition Program for Women, Infants, and Children (WIC): www.fns.usda.gov/wic/about-wic.

BREECH AND BABY'S POSITIONS IN UTERO

Breech Version: How a Doula or Partner May Help. www.pennysimkin.com/ download

Evidence Based Birth: www.evidence-basedbirth.com.

Simkin, Penny, and Ruth Ancheta. 2017. *The Labor Progress Handbook: Early Interventions to Prevent and Treat Dystocia*, 4th ed.

Spinning Babies: www.spinningbabies.com.

What Your Baby's Position in the Womb Means: www.healthline.com/health/ pregnancy/baby-positions-in-womb.

CESAREAN DELIVERY

Childbirth Connection. 2016. *What Every Woman Needs to Know About Cesarean Birth*. National Partnership for Women & Families. www.nationalpartnership.org/research-library/ maternal-health/ what-every-pregnant-woman-needs-to-know-about-cesarean-section.pdf.

Childbirth Connection. 2016. *Why is the C-Section Rate so High?* National Partnership for Women & Families. www. nationalpartnership.org/research-library/maternal-health/ why-is-the-c-section-rate-so-high.pdf.

Haelle, Tara. 2018. "Your Biggest C-Section Risk May Be Your Hospital." *Consumer Reports*. ww.consumerreports.org/c-section/biggest-c-section-risk-may-be-your-hospital.

CIRCUMCISION

American Academy of Pediatrics. 2012. Policy statement. "Circumcision Policy Statement." Task Force on Circumcision. pediatrics.aappublications.org/ content/pediatrics/130/3/585.full.pdf.

Canadian Paediatric Society. 2015. "Newborn Male Circumcision." Position Statement. www.cps.ca/en/documents/ position/circumcision.

Kass, Elias. 2018. "Circumcision." https:// drdadsays.com/2018/02/09/circumcision.

COMFORT ADVICE AND AIDS FOR CHILDBIRTH

Pregnancy and Labor Ice Pack: www. pennysimkin.com/shop/pregnancy-and-labor-ice-pack.

Simkin, Penny. 2007. "Comfort in Labor." Available at no cost from www. childbirthconnection.org/pdfs/comfort-in-labor-simkin.pdf.

Simkin, Penny. 2008. *Comfort Measures for Childbirth*. DVD. www.pennysimkin.com.

CORD-BLOOD STORAGE

American Academy of Pediatrics. 2007. Policy Statement. "Cord Blood Banking for Potential Future Transplantation." pediatrics.aappublications.org/ content/pediatrics/119/1/165.full.pdf.

KidsHealth. 2015. The Nemours Foundation. "Cord-Blood Banking." kidshealth. org/en/parents/cord-blood.html

CUTTING THE UMBILICAL CORD

Bakalar, Nicholas. 2011. New Cochrane Review. "Childbirth: Benefits Seen in Clamping the Cord Later." The *New York Times*. www.nytimes.com/2011/11/29/health/research/delay-in-clamping-umbilical-cord-has-benefits-months-later.html.

Science & Sensibility. 2017. *New Cochrane Review*. "Delayed Cord Clamping Likely Beneficial for Healthy Term Newborns." www.scienceandsensibility.org/blog/new-cochrane-review-delayed- cord-clamping-likely-beneficial-for-healthy-term-newborns.

Simkin, Penny. 2012. *Penny Simkin on Delayed Cord Clamping*. www.youtube.com/watch?v=W3RywNup2CM.

FUSSY, CRYING BABIES

Brazelton, T. Berry, and Joshua D. Sparrow. 2003. *Calming Your Fussy Baby: The Brazelton Way.*

Karp, Harvey. 2003. *The Happiest Baby on the Block.* (Also available on DVD.)

Nugent, Kevin. 2011. *Your Baby Is Speaking to You: A Visual Guide to the Amazing Behaviors of Your Newborn and Growing Baby.*

Pantley, Elizabeth. 2002. *The No-Cry Sleep Solution: Gentle Ways to Help Your Baby Sleep Through the Night.*

Sears, William, and Martha Sears. 1996. *The Fussy Baby Book: Parenting Your High-Need Child from Birth to Age Five.*

Plooij, Frans X. 2017. *The Wonder Weeks: How to Stimulate Your Baby's Mental Development and Help Him Turn His 10 Predictable, Great, Fussy Phases into Magical Leaps Forward.* Also has an outstanding app for baby milestones: www.thewonderweeks.com.

GENDER NEUTRAL INFORMATION

Canadian Midwives Trans Inclusivity Statement: www.canadianmidwives.org/2015/09/25/trans-inclusivity-statement.

MANA Statement on Gender Inclusive Language: www.mana.org/healthcare-policy/position-statement-on-gender-inclusive-language.

The *New York Times* Gender Neutral Glossary: www.nytimes.com/2015/02/08/education/a-gender-neutral-glossary.html.

GESTATIONAL DIABETES

Diabetic Mommy: www.diabeticmommy.com.

Geil, Patti Bazel, Patricia Geil, and Laura Hieronymus. 2003. *101 Tips for a Healthy Pregnancy with Diabetes.*

GRIEF AND TRAUMATIC BIRTH

Church, Lisa, and Ann H. Prescott. 2004. *Hope Is Like the Sun: Finding Hope and Healing After Miscarriage, Stillbirth, or Infant Death.*

Douglas, Ann, John R. Sussman, and Deborah Davis. 2000. *Trying Again: A Guide to Pregnancy After Miscarriage, Stillbirth, and Infant Loss.*

Faces of Loss: A place for mothers to share their story of miscarriage, stillbirth, and infant loss. www.facesofloss.com.

HopeXchange Publishing: www.hopexchange.com (on miscarriage, stillbirth, and infant death).

Kitzinger, Sheila. 2006. *Birth Crisis.*

Madsen, Lynn. 1994. *Rebounding from Childbirth: Toward Emotional Recovery.*

Now I Lay Me Down To Sleep: free remembrance photography services for stillbirth: www.nowilaymedowntosleep.org.

P.A.T.T.C.h (Prevention and Treatment of Traumatic Childbirth). *The Traumatic Birth Prevention and Resource Guide,* a collection of reflections written by many of the PATTCh Board members, explains the components of traumatic birth, increases awareness, and promotes prevention. www.pattch.org/resource-guide.

Schweibert, Pat, and Paul Kirk. 2012. *When Hello Means Goodbye*, 3rd revision.

Simkin, Penny, and Phyllis Klaus. 2004. *When Survivors Give Birth: Understanding and Healing the Effects of Early Sexual Abuse on Childbearing Women.*

HYPNOSIS FOR BIRTH

Mongan, Marie. 2015. *HypnoBirthing: The Mongan Method: A Natural Approach to a Safe, Easier, More Comfortable Birthing*, 4th ed.

O'Neill, Michelle Leclaire. 2000. *Hypnobirthing: The Original Method: Mindful Pregnancy and Easy Labor Using the Leclaire Childbirth Method.*

Tuschhoff, Kerry. "Hypnobabies Home Study Course." www.hypnobabies.com.

LABOR SUPPORT TOOLS AND TENS UNIT PURCHASE

Hutch. An App for Comfort and Progress in Labor (Brief videos showing dozens of techniques to use for pain and slow progress [without and with an epidural]) www.pennysimkin.com

Apollo Massage Roller: www.amazon.com.

TENS unit rentals/sales in Europe (also ships to U.S.): www.babycaretens.com.

TENS unit rentals in the U.S. and Canada: www.midwiferysupplies.ca/products/elle-tens-machine. (Many doulas have TENS units available for loan or low-cost rental.)

TENS unit sales in the U.S.: www.sharonmuza.com.

LOCATING A BIRTH OR POSTPARTUM DOULA

DONA International: www.dona.org.

DoulaMatch.net: www.doulamatch.net.

Klaus, Marshall H., John H. Kennell, and Phyllis H. Klaus. 2012. *The Doula Book: How a Trained Labor Companion Can Help You Have a Shorter, Easier, and Healthier Birth.*

MEAL TRAINS AND CHORE SIGN-UPS

CareCalendar: www.carecalendar.org.

Lotsa Helping Hands: www.lotsahelpinghands.com.

Take Them a Meal: www.takethemameal.com.

NEWBORN SCREENING TESTS

March of Dimes. "Newborn Screening Tests for Your Baby." www.marchofdimes.org/newborn-screening-tests-for-your-baby.aspx.

Screening tests by state: www.babysfirsttest.org/newborn screening/states.

PELVIC FLOOR SELF-ASSESSMENT PAMPHLET

Dr. April Bolding: www.aprilbolding.com.

PLACENTA ENCAPSULATION

Dekker, Rebecca. 2017. "The Evidence on Placenta Encapsulation." www.evidencebasedbirth.com/evidence-on-placenta encapsulation.

Find placenta specialists and other questions to ask: www.findplacentaencapsulation.com.

POSTPARTUM DEPRESSION ONLINE SUPPORT

Postpartum Support International (PSI) online support: www.postpartum.net/learn-more/help-for-moms.

Solace for Mothers: www.solaceformothers.org.

POSTPARTUM DOULAS

Kelleher, Jacqueline. 2002. *Nurturing the Family: The Guide for Postpartum Doulas.*

Pascali Bonaro, Debra. 2014. *Nurturing Beginnings: Guide to Postpartum Care for Doulas and Community Outreach Workers.*

Webber, Salle. 2012. *The Gentle Art of Newborn Family Care: A Guide for Postpartum Doulas and Caregivers.*

POSTPARTUM EMOTIONS AND DEPRESSION

Postpartum Support International (PSI). Dedicated to helping women suffering from perinatal mood and anxiety disorders, including postpartum depression. www.postpartum.net.

PREGNANCY APPS FOR TRACKING FETAL MOVEMENTS AND CONTRACTIONS

Full Term: www.fulltermapp.com.

Ovia Pregnancy (and others): www.ovuline.com.

Sprout Pregnancy: www.sprout-apps.com.

PREMATURITY AND KANGAROO CARE

Bergman, Nils M.D., Ph.D, and Jill Bergman. www.kangaroomothercare.com.

Bradford, Nikki, Jonathan Hellman, Sharyn Gibbins, and Sandra Lousada. 2003. *Your Premature Baby: The First Five Years.*

March of Dimes: www.marchofdimes.org.

Sears, William, Robert Sears, James Sears, and Martha Sears. 2004. *The Premature Baby Book: Everything You Need to Know About Your Premature Baby from Birth to Age One.*

PREPARING OLDER CHILDREN FOR THE BIRTH OF A SIBLING

Overend, Jenni, and Julie Vivas. 1999. *Welcome with Love.*

Simkin, Penny, Janet Whalley, Ann Keppler, Janelle Durham, and April Bolding. 2016. *Pregnancy, Childbirth, and the Newborn: The Complete Guide,* 5th ed. (chapter 16).

Simkin, Penny (producer and writer), and Walter Zamojski (videographer and film editor). 2013. *There's a Baby: A Children's Film About a New Baby.* DVD for children (shows a birth). www.pennysimkin.com.

PROPER CARE OF THE UNCIRCUMCISED PENIS

Most comprehensive infant-care books contain a section on this topic.

WebMD. 2017. "How to Care for Your Baby Boy's Penis." www.webmd.com/ parenting/baby/tc/your-newborn-boys-genitals-care-of-penis.

SINGING TO BABY BEFORE AND AFTER BIRTH

Chamberlain, David. 2013. *Windows to the Womb: Revealing the Conscious Baby from Conception to Birth.*

Fink, Cathy, and Marcy Marxer. 2011. *Sing to Your Baby.* (CD/playbook).

Simkin, Penny. 2013. Singing to the Baby. www.youtube.com/watch?v=gsdE-K6OxucA.

VAGINAL BIRTH AFTER CESAREAN (VBAC)

Churchill, Helen. 2010. *Vaginal Birth After Caesarean.*

International Cesarean Awareness Network: www.ican-online.org.

American College of Obstetricians and Gynecologists. 2017. Practice Bulletin No. 184: Vaginal Birth After Cesarean Delivery. *Obstetrics & Gynecology* 130 (5): 1167–1169. https://journals.lww.com/greenjournal/Fulltext2017/11000/Practice_Bulletin_No_184_Vaginal_Birth_After.51.aspx.

VBAC FACTS:

www.vbacfacts.com.
www.vbac.com.

VITAMIN K

American Academy of Pediatrics. Policy
Statement. "Controversies Concerning
Vitamin K and the Newborn." http://
pediatrics.aappublications.org/con-
tent/112/1/191.full.
Canadian Paediatric Society. Position
Statement. "Routine administration of
vitamin K to newborns." www.cps.ca/
en/ documents/position/administra-
tion-vitamin-K-newborns.

WATERBIRTH INFORMATION, TUB RENTAL, AND SALES

AquaDoula: www.aquadoula.com.
Waterbirth International: www.waterbirth.org.
Waterbirth Solutions:
www.waterbirthsolutions.com.
Your Water Birth: www.yourwaterbirth.com.

Index

A

Abdominal lifting, 95, 97
Active labor, 31, 36, 37–40
Active relaxation, 55, 58
Acupressure, 100
Acyclovir, 127
Afterpains, 169
Amnioinfusion, 113
Amniotic fluid, 22, 67, 104, 105,
    111, 112, 152, 160–161
Antibiotics, 22, 103–104, 135, 141
Antiviral medication, 127
Apgar score, 49, 52, 106, 158, 162
Apps, timing contractions, 27
Arrested labor, 129, 150
Arrest of active labor, 129–130
Artificial rupture of the mem-
    branes (AROM), 111–113, 114
Asynclitism, 93
Attention focusing, 59–60, 100
Auscultation, 111

B

Baby
    bathing, 165–166
    bowel movements, 165
    choosing a caregiver for, 14–15
    circumcision of, 167–168
    common procedures for care
        of newborn, 160–164
    feeding, 166
    fussy and crying, 177
    gestational diabetes mellitus
        and, 126
    importance of holding and
        cuddling, 164–165
    physical exam and assess-
        ment of, 165
    screening tests for newborn,
        166–167
Baby (unborn). See Fetus
Baby blues, 173–175
Baby care and safety class, 14
Backache/back pain, 19, 21, 96
Back, laying on with legs drawn
    up (position), 76
Back massage, 81–82

Bag of waters, breaking before
    labor begins, 22–23. See also
    Ruptured membranes
Baths, 77–80, 94, 112, 165–166
Bed, labor in, 99
Bedrest, 124
Bilirubin levels, 136–137, 163
Birth ball, 66, 68, 71, 72, 81, 98
Birthing stage of labor, 29, 43–50,
    53, 57–58, 96, 98–99
Birth in water, 79–80
Birth options, in Birth Plan, 12
Birth partner
    being reachable, 9
    characteristics of being a
        good, 16
    feelings of, after childbirth, 175
    holding and cuddling baby
        after birth, 164–165
    reaction to rapid labor, 90
    during recovery and bonding
        stage, 52
    during resting phase, 45
    role during cesarean birth,
        155–157
    role of, 16
    roles during slow-to-start
        labor, 93–94
    role when laboring person has
        a narcotic, 138–139
    role when using epidurals, 140
    Take Charge routine used by,
        86–88
Birth partner, help from
    during active labor, 36–37,
        39–40
    during an arrest of labor, 130
    with bleeding during labor,
        128
    during complicated late
        pregnancies and labor,
        123–124
    with complications during the
        placental stage, 133
    with complications with the
        newborn, 134
    during crowning and birth
        phase, 49–50
    with delay in labor, 99
    during descent phase, 47–48
    during early labor, 34–36
    gestational diabetes and, 126

with herpes lesion, 127
with labor rituals, 57
during placental stage of
    labor, 51
practicing and using relax-
    ation with pregnant/
    laboring person, 58, 59
during prelabor, 30–31
with a prolapsed cord, 131, 132
during transition phase, 42
Birth Plan, 11–13, 182–185
Birth trauma/injury, 136
Bleeding after birth, 128–129
Bleeding during labor, 127–128
Bleeding, excessive postpartum,
    133
Blood
    cord, 12, 50, 161, 163
    placental, 153, 161–162
Blood pressure, 139, 141. See also
    High blood pressure
Blood sugar, 126, 136, 163
Blood tests, for newborn, 163
Blue feelings, after childbirth,
    173–175
Body temperature, newborn, 135
Bowel movements
    of baby, 165
    of birthing parent after birth,
        170
    soft, 21
Braxton Hicks contractions,
    21, 23
Breast milk, 134–135
Breath holding, 64, 65–66
Breathing problems, in newborn,
    135
Breech presentation, 26, 104, 112,
    131, 150

C

Caregiver(s). See also Midwives
    during active labor, 38–39
    during birthing stage of labor,
        43–44
    for cesarean births, 151
    choosing for baby, 14–15
    during crowning and birth
        phase, 49
    during descent phase, 47
    discussing self-induction
        measures with, 91

during early labor, 33
essential observations during labor by, 104–106
during placental stage of labor, 50
preferences regarding medical intervention, 106–107
during prelabor, 30
questions about medical interventions and tests for, 101–102
during recovery and bonding stage, 52
during resting phase, 45
during transition phase, 41
visiting before labor, 4–5
when to call, 32
Cat-cow pose, 9, 10
Cervix
centimeters of length, 25
change in position of, 24
dilation of, 20, 31, 36, 37
slow-to-start labor and, 92
softening of, 24
thinning and shortening of, 25
Cesarean birth, 13, 130, 147–157, 159, 170–171
Chair, sitting and rocking in a, 71
Chores, household, 178–179
Circumcision, 167–168
Clamping, of umbilical cord, 50, 153, 161–162
Clamps, with cesarean births, 171
Classes
baby care and safety, 14
parent infant, 14
Code word, 42, 88, 146, 147
Colostrum, 13, 135, 166
Comfort measures. See also Relaxation; Rhythmic breathing
during active labor, 40
attention focusing, 59–60
for backache during labor, 96
baths and showers, 77–80
changes in movement or position, 66–76
for laboring in bed, 100
massage and touch, 80–85
with music and sound, 85
for perineum after birth, 169–170

for pushing (bearing down), 64–66
visualization, 60–61
Commode, sitting on a, 70
Complications related to labor
arrest of active labor, 129–130
excessive bleeding, 127–129
fetal heart rate problems, 132–133
gestational diabetes mellitus (GDM), 125–126
herpes lesion, 127
high blood pressure, 124–125
with the newborn, 134–136
during the placental stage, 133
premature labor, 124
prolapsed cord, 131–132
Contractions
after birth, 159
afterpains, 169
Braxton-Hicks, 21, 23
during early labor, 33
in first stage of labor, 31
nipple stimulation for bringing on or intensifying, 91–92
nonprogressing, 21, 23–24, 26, 29
prelabor, 17, 30
premature labor and, 22
progressing, 21, 25, 30
timing, 26–27
Cord blood, 12, 50
Counterpressure, 100
Cramps, 21, 50
Crowning and birth phase, 48–50
Crying baby, 177

D
Dangle position, 46, 48, 75–76, 98, 99, 122
Death of a baby, 137
Depression, postpartum, 173–175
Descent phase of second stage of labor, 25, 26, 45–48, 98–99
Diabetes (pregnant person), 104, 115, 149, 150. See also Gestational diabetes mellitus (GDM)
Dilation stage of labor, 29, 31–43
Directed pushing, 65–66, 122
Distracting activities, 34, 55, 94

Doctor. See Caregiver(s); Obstetricians
DONA International, 8
Doppler ultrasound, 39, 79
Doula(s), 5–8, 35–36, 151, 172, 178
DoulaMatch.net, 7, 8
Dystocia (arrest of active labor), 129–130

E
Early labor, 26, 31, 32–36, 55, 60, 94
Early Labor Record, 33, 189
Eclampsia, 125
Elective induction, 90, 116–117
Electronic fetal monitor(ing) (EFM), 38, 39, 99, 100, 104, 108–111, 115, 117, 118
Emotions, 16, 19, 29, 37, 86, 130, 142, 173–175
Encapsulation, of the placenta, 159–160
Epidurals, 44, 46, 51, 66, 98, 99, 107, 129, 130, 138, 139–142, 140
Episiotomy, 12, 38, 49, 118–120, 158
Excessive bleeding, 127–129, 133. See also Hemorrhage
Exercises, 9–10
Eye medication, for newborn, 162

F
"False" labor, 23–24
Feeding, of baby, 164, 177–178
Fetal heart rate problems, 132
Fetal movement counting, 150, 188
Fetal scalp stimulation test, 111
Fever, 141
First stage of labor, 29, 31–43, 53
5-1-1 rule, 33
Flexion, 25
Foot massage, 84–85
Forceful pushing, avoiding, 64
Forceps, 47, 66, 99, 121–122, 130, 142
Formula feeding, 135, 166
4-1-1 rule, 33
Fourth stage of labor, 29, 51–52
Fundal massage, 159

G

General analgesia, 143
General anesthesia, 107, 108, 138, 143–144
Gestational diabetes mellitus (GDM), 125–126
Gestational hypertension (GH), 125
Group B streptococcus, 22–23, 103, 160
Grunt pushes, 64

H

Hand massage, 83–84
Hands-and-knees position, 41, 46, 47, 48, 71, 95. *See also* Open knee-chest position
Hands-and-knees rocking, 9, 10, 76, 122
Hearing screening test, 166–167
HELLP syndrome, 125
Hemorrhage, 128–129, 144, 150, 168
Herpes lesion, 127
High blood pressure, 99, 104, 115, 124–125
Home birth, 29, 30, 33, 34, 36, 77, 172, 187
Hospital
    arriving and admitting at too early, 29, 33
    average stay in, 172
    preregistration at, 5
    when to call, 32
    when to go to the, 33–34
Household chores, 178–179
Hypnosis, 100

I

Incontinence, 10, 149
Induced labor. *See* Labor induction
Infection
    AROM and, 112
    baths and, 79, 112
    electronic fetal monitoring and, 110
    Group B Strep, 103–104
    in newborn, 135
    within the uterus, 22–23
Inhalation analgesia, 143
Intrauterine pressure catheter, 108, 110, 113, 130
IV (intravenous) fluids, 100, 103, 104, 107–108, 129

J

Jaundice, 126, 136–137, 161, 163

K

Kangaroo care, 135
Kegel (pelvic floor contraction) exercise, 9, 10–11, 170
Key Questions for Informed Decision-Making, 101–102
Kneeling lunge movement, 69

L

Labor
    bag of waters breaking before beginning of, 22–23
    comfort measures for. *See* Comfort measures
    complications related to. *See* Complications related to labor
    dilation (first) stage of, 31–43
    essential observations during, 104–106
    factors influencing length of, 19
    "false," 23–24
    first (dilation) stage of, 29, 31–43, 53
    fourth (recovery) stage of, 29, 51–52
    getting ready for, 4–11
    placental (third) stage of, 29, 50–51
    positions and movements for, 66–76
    prelabor *vs.*, 17–18
    progression of, 24–26
    rapid, 89–90
    second (birthing) stage of, 29, 43–50, 53, 57–58, 96, 98–99
    signs of, 20–22
    slow-to-start, 92–99
    step-by-step process of, 17
    third stage of, 29, 50–51
    unpredictability of, 28
Labor induction, 18, 90–92
    disadvantages of, 115–116

GBS screening and, 103
    methods for, 114–115
    nonmedical reasons for, 116–118
Labor options, in Birth Plan, 12
Labor-stimulating measures, 90–92, 94
Lacerations, 129, 133
Lap squatting, 46, 48, 75, 98, 99
Latent phase (early labor). *See* Early labor
Light breathing, 62, 63
Local anesthesia, 118, 142, 143, 158, 167, 168
Lochia, 129, 169
LOP (left occiput posterior), 97, 98
Low blood sugar, 126, 136
Lunge, 6, 41, 69, 97

M

Mantras, 59–60
Massage, 80–85, 100
Meconium, 22, 105, 112, 113, 132, 160, 165
Medical induction, 90
Medical interventions, 29. *See also* Labor induction; Pain medications
    during active labor, 38
    amnioinfusion, 113
    artificial rupture of the membranes, 111–113
    conditions influencing, during labor, 106–107
    during early labor, 33
    electronic fetal monitoring. *See* Electronic fetal monitor(ing) (EFM)
    episiotomies, 118–120
    forceps delivery, 121–122
    IV fluids, 107–108
    questions for informed decision-making with, 101–102
    vacuum extraction, 120–121
Medications. *See also* Antibiotics; Pain medications
    antiviral, 127
    blood pressure, 125
    with cesarean births, 154, 156
    eye, for newborn, 162

sleep-inducing, 154
Mental ritual, 59–60
Midwives, 36, 79, 80, 95, 104,
118, 172.
Moaning, 40, 56, 57, 61–62
Modified directed pushing, 66
Molding of baby's head, 25, 26, 48
Mucus discharge, 21

N

Narcotics, 129, 135, 138–139, 156
Nesting urge, 21
Newborn
    caregiver observations of, 106
    common procedures in care
        of, 160–164
    complications with the,
        134–137
    death of, 137
    herpes in, 127
    immediately after the birth,
        158
    suctioning nose and mouth of,
        160–161
Nipple stimulation, 91–92, 159
Nitrous oxide, 143
Nonprogressing contractions, 21,
    23–24, 26, 29
Nonstress test, 104, 150
Nurse. *See* Caregiver(s)

O

OA (occiput anterior) position,
    10, 19, 25, 32, 96
Obstetricians, 38–39
Open knee-chest position, 10, 56,
    72, 95, 131, 132
OP (occiput posterior) position,
    19, 93, 96
Orgasm, 92
OT (occiput transverse) position,
    19, 96
Oxytocin, 46, 51, 52, 78, 91, 92, 99,
    110, 112, 115, 130, 141, 153, 159

P

Packing for hospital or birth
    center, 9, 181, 186
Pain during labor
    causes of, 53
    decreasing, 54–55. *See also*
        Comfort measures

suffering *vs.*, 53–54
Pain medications, 42. *See also*
    Epidurals
    active labor and, 37, 130
    in birth plan, 12
    general analgesia and anes-
        thesia, 143–144
    knowing how the birthing
        person feels about,
        144–147
    knowing preferences for, 54
    labor in bed and, 99
    overview, 138
    suggested during difficult
        labor, 88
    supporting during active
        labor, 37
    take-charge routine and, 88
    transition phase and, 42
Pain Medications Preference
    Scale (PMPS), 144–147
Parenting groups, 15
Parents
    getting enough sleep, 176–177
    meals for new, 178
    receiving help from others, 172
Passive relaxation, 55, 58
Pelvic floor contractions (Kegel),
    9, 10–11, 170
Pelvic rocking, 9, 10, 95, 97
Perineal care, 12
Perineal care, in birth plan, 12
Perineal massage, 12, 48, 128
Perineum, 12, 45, 47, 48, 52
    care of, after vaginal birth,
        169–183
    comfort measures for sore,
        169–170
    episiotomy and, 118–119, 120
Phototherapy, 136–137
Pitocin, 115, 117, 130, 133, 140,
    141, 159
Placenta, 127, 129, 133, 154, 161–162
Placental abruption, 127, 128
Placental encapsulation, 159–160
Placental stage of labor, 29,
    50–51, 133
Placenta previa, 128
Plan B, in Birth Plan, 11, 13
Planned rituals, 55–56
Platoon sleeping, 177
Position(s)

of baby in uterus, 19, 93, 96,
    150
    to change the baby's position,
        97–99
    for labor and birth, 47, 48,
        68–76
    stimulating labor, 95
Positive signs of labor, 20, 21
Possible signs of labor, 20, 21
Postpartum bleeding, 133
Postpartum care options, in Birth
    Plan, 12
Postpartum hemorrhage, 128–129
Post-term births, 18
Preeclampsia, 125, 150
Pregnancy, birth partner's role
    during last weeks of, 4–15
Prelabor, 29–31
Prelabor contractions, 21, 23–24
Prelabor, labor *vs.*, 17–18
Prelabor signs, 20, 21
Premature (preterm) births, 13,
    18, 22, 124, 136
Presentation, 19, 93, 104, 131, 150
Progressing contractions, 21,
    25, 30
Prolapsed cord, 23, 112, 131–132,
    144, 150
Prolonged bedrest, 124
Prolonged labor, 115, 120, 129–130,
    136. *See also* Slow-to-start
    labor
Protracted labor, 129
Pushing, 45–46
    avoiding forceful, 64
    comfort measures for, 64–66
    directed, 65–66
    with epidurals, 141–142
    modified directed, 66
    self-directed, 65
    spontaneous bearing down,
        65

R

Rapid labor, 20, 89–90
Recovery and bonding (fourth)
    stage of labor, 29, 51–52
Rectal pain, 142
Relaxation, 36, 42, 55, 58–59, 94,
    100. *See also* Rhythmic
    breathing

Resting phase of second stage of labor, 44–45
Retained placenta, 129, 133
Rhythmic breathing, 35, 54, 56, 58, 61–64, 100, 153
Rhythm/rhythmic ritual, 36, 38, 40, 42, 45–46, 56
Rituals, labor, 55–57.
Rocking in a chair, 71
Ruptured membranes, 22–23, 79, 92, 114
    artificial rupture of the membranes (AROM), 111–112

S

Screening tests, newborn, 166–167
Second stage of labor. *See* Birthing stage of labor
Self-directed pushing, 65
Self-induction, 90–92
Semiprone position, 73, 98
Semisitting position, 66, 67, 70
Sexually transmitted diseases (STDs), 167
Sexual stimulation, self-induction through, 92
"Show," 21
Showers, 77–78, 94
Side lying, 46, 47, 64, 73, 97, 98, 171
Signs of labor, 20
Sitting upright position, 67, 70
Skin-to-skin contact, 51, 52, 135, 153, 158, 164
Sleep (newborn), 177–178
Sleep deprivation (parents), 176
Slow breathing, 62, 63, 94, 95
Slow dancing, 40, 57, 68, 95, 97
Slow-to-start labor, 92–99
Special-care nursery, 134, 156
Spinal blocks, 138, 139–140
Spontaneous bearing down, 64, 65, 66
Spontaneous rituals, 36, 38, 56, 100
Squatting, 9–10, 74, 75
Standing and leaning position, 68
Standing lunge movement, 69
Standing position, 67
Stillbirth, 13, 115, 126
Stitches, 119, 154, 158–159, 171
Suctioning baby's nose and mouth, 106, 153, 160–161

T

Take Charge routine, 42, 57, 86–88, 100
Telemetry monitors, 79, 100, 109, 111
Tests
    blood, of newborn, 163
    fetal scalp stimulation, 111
    hearing screening, 166–167
    late-pregnancy, 103–104
    nonstress, 104, 150
    questions for informed decision-making with, 101–102
    screening, for newborn, 166–167
Third stage of labor, 29, 50–51
"3 to 6 phase," 36
Three Rs. *See* Relaxation; Rhythm/rhythmic ritual; Rituals, labor
Timing contractions, 26–27
Tocodynamometer, 108, 110
Tocophobia, 148
Toilet, sitting on a, 70
Touch and massage, 80–85
Toxemia, 125
Transcutaneous electrical nerve stimulation (TENS), 96, 100
Transition phase, 41–42

U

Ultrasonography, 104
Umbilical cord, 50, 51
    AROM and, 112
    blood, 12, 50, 161, 163
    caring for, after birth, 166
    clamping and cutting the, 50, 153, 161–162
    prolapsed, 23, 131–132
Urge to push, 41, 42, 43, 44, 45–46, 64–65

V

Vacuum extraction/extractor, 7, 38, 47, 66, 99, 120–121, 122, 130, 136, 142, 153
Vaginal birth after cesarean, 150–151
Vaginal discharge, 169
Vaginal exams, 22, 47
Vaginal pain, 142

Valacyclovir, 127
Versed, 154
Vertex, 19
Visualization, 60–61
Vital signs, checked after birth, 159
Vitamin K, 162

W

Walking
    during labor, 67
    self-induction through, 92
    stimulating labor with, 95
Warming unit, 51, 163–164
Water births, 79–80
Water leaks, 21, 22
Water temperature, bath or shower, 78, 79, 94

Z

Zofran, 154